PRO-NURSE HANDBOOK

**Designed for the Nurse
who wants to** ~~survive~~ *thrive*
professionally

Melodie Chenevert, author of *Pro-Nurse Handbook* and *STAT: Special Techniques in Assertiveness Training for Women in the Health Professions,* is a consultant and specialist in continuing education.

Her latest major project was setting up an entire school of nursing from scratch on the Oregon coast. Fragments of that experience appear in this book.

She received her diploma (1963) from Methodist-Kahler School of Nursing in Rochester, Minnesota; her bachelor's (1966) and master's (1968) degrees from the University of Washington-Seattle with a clinical specialty in psychiatric nursing; and an MA in journalism (1978) from the University of Wisconsin-Madison. She has worked as a staff nurse and play therapist/child mental health clinician and for several years was an instructor in psychiatric nursing at the University of Wisconsin.

PRO-NURSE HANDBOOK

Designed for the Nurse who wants to survive *thrive* professionally

Melodie Chenevert

Illustrated

The C. V. Mosby Company

ST. LOUIS · TORONTO · PRINCETON   1985

To Gary, Eric, Ryan, and Panzer

Editor: Nancy L. Mullins
Assistant editor: Bess Arends, Maureen Slaten
Editing supervisor: Judi Wolken
Manuscript editor: Melissa Neves
Book design: Jeanne Genz
Cover design: Tilford Smith
Production: Barbara Merritt

Printed in the United States of America

The C.V. Mosby Company
11830 Westline Industrial Drive, St. Louis, Missouri 63146

Library of Congress Cataloging in Publication Data

Chenevert, Melodie, 1941–
   Pro-nurse handbook.

   Includes index.
   1. Nurses—Psychology.   2. Nursing—Social aspects.
3. Leadership.   I. Title.   [DNLM: 1. Nursing.
2. Career Mobility.   3. Interprofessional Relations.
WY 16 C518p]
RT86.C48   1985   610.73   84-20573
ISBN 0-8016-1156-3

VT/VH/VH   9   8   7   6   5   4   3   2   1   05/D/645

Contents

Prologue

Out of the blue . . .

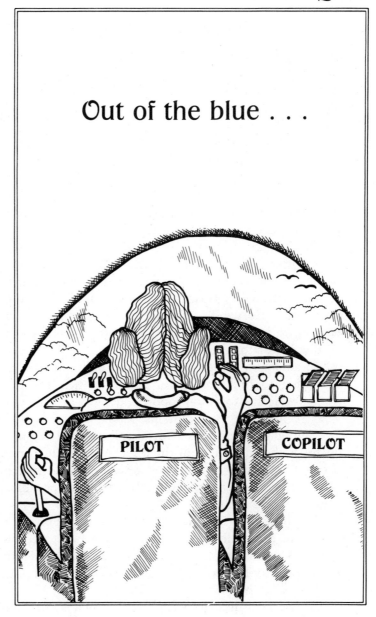

Being admitted to the hospital is much like boarding an airplane. The cost is sky high. Once on board you must relinquish control to the crew. You must trust their judgment, follow their schedules, and adhere to their rules. Whether passenger or patient, you pray for a safe landing at the desired destination.

Your contact on the plane is almost exclusively with the stewardess. She greets you, seats you, comforts and feeds you. In the hospital the nurse performs similar functions. Perhaps that's why she is so easily mistaken for a "stewardess."

Pilots, like doctors, are essentially inaccessible. Occasionally their voices boom over the loudspeaker announcing the speed, altitude, weather conditions, and estimated time of arrival.

Over the years passengers have come to rely on the stewardess for their comfort and on the pilot for their safety. In much the same fashion, patients have come to rely on the nurse for their comfort and on the doctor for their safety.

In an analogy between a hospital unit and an airplane, it is not surprising to find the doctor assuming he's the pilot. Whenever analogies of this sort are proposed, doctors assume the key position. They see themselves as captains, kings, or quarterbacks.

The hospital administrator also leaps to the conclusion that the doctor is the equivalent of the pilot. He sees doctors, like pilots, as necessary. He sees nurses, like stewardesses, as nice but not necessary. Nonessential nurses: interchangeable, disposable. Hospital policies reflect his view.

The nurse also assumes the doctor is in the pilot's seat. She scurries about the cabin smiling and serving. When turbulence occurs, she goes forward to the cockpit. To her horror she finds it empty. She slides into the pilot's seat, not out of choice but out of necessity.

She is catapulted from stewardess to pilot. Hearing the passengers ring for service, she is confused. Which is *real* nursing? Cabin or cockpit? She shuttles back and forth trying to do both jobs at once.

Her confusion is compounded by space-age doctors who beam aboard at irregular and unpredictable intervals. They materialize for a few moments, demand to know why the nurse is in the pilot's seat, and order her to return to the cabin where she belongs. The nurse complies.

Before long the plane goes into another tailspin, and once again she finds herself in the pilot's seat. She sits uneasily. She never wanted to steer. She just wanted to serve. Yet in real life the nurse is more analogous to the pilot than the doctor is.

Think about it. In this analogy the doctor cannot be the pilot for one simple reason. He is not on board. Actually, the doctor is more analogous to ground control. Essential but absent.

Nurses know getting in touch with ground control is difficult at best. The communication system is unreliable. Messages are garbled. Even when contact is established, nurses often get nothing but static. (As long as doctors and administrators insist on flying by remote control, they would be wise to uprade the communication system and stop downgrading nurses.)

A veteran pilot quipped that flying is 95 percent boredom and 5 percent sheer terror. Fortunately for the pilot, his compensation is not based on 95 percent of the flying he does. His compensation is based on the 5 percent he hopes he doesn't have to do. He is compensated for those times when he must override automation and exercise all his training, skill, judgment, and experience to correct errors, minimize complications, and avert catastrophes.

Nursing, like flying, is 95 percent routine and predictable. Almost automatic. But nursing also has its 5 percent sheer terror. Unlike the pilot, unfortunately, a nurse's compensation is based on the routine and predictable (cabin duties). She is not compensated for her training, skill, judgment, or experience. She is not compensated for correcting errors, minimizing complications, and averting catastrophes (cockpit duties).

Imagine saying to a pilot, "Look, you and I both know that superb engineering has made flying almost automatic. Sure we need an expert's touch for takeoffs and landings, but in between you've got a lot of time on your hands. Once you're sure the plane is on course, go back into the cabin and serve refreshments. Make sure everyone's happy. But keep one eye on the instrument panel just in case something goes wrong."

Any pilot would tell you to take a flying leap. Pilots know how to provide service without being subservient. Nurses must learn to do the same. It's a matter of survival.

Science and technology have gifted us with gizmos, gadgets, and all sorts of mechanical miracles. Without the proper human connection, however, they are utterly worthless.

Reading meters, graphs, and gauges takes skill. Reading patients takes even more skill. Nurses must be able to do both. We must monitor the machinery and mind the patients.

We must be able to detect a subtle slowing of activity, a grimace, an involuntary twitch, a faint odor, a slight variation in respiration. We must read between the lines. We must hear the unspoken word.

Many changes, most too minuscule for the unskilled eye or ear, signal the need for minor corrections. Failure to make those minor corrections can lead to major malfunctions. For airplane passengers the results range from discomfort to death. The same is true for hospital patients. It matters not whether the error is caused by inexperience, ignorance, or inattention. The result is the same.

Now, from out of the blue, come DRGs and other cost-containment policies forcing hospitals to carry full loads of complex patients from sickness to wellness in record time. Nurses fear the result will be roughly equivalent to having patients "deplane" at 1000 feet. The knowledge that we brought them down safely the first 34,000 feet is small consolation.

If our patients are to survive, nurses will have to stay in the cockpit where we can see clearly and effect safe landings. Cabin-bound nurses can't set the course or change directions. They just get taken for a ride.

It's precisely because we have spent more time in the cabin than in the cockpit that our profession is in a crash-and-burn configuration. Unless we assume command, we may not survive. Unless we learn to command well, we will not thrive.

The *Pro-Nurse Handbook* is designed to help you pilot your own craft. Don't keep flying by the seat of your pants. Learn to fly first class.

Jettison your stewardess complex, strap yourself into the pilot's seat, and prepare for turbulence. There may be some rough weather ahead, but remember, you can't reach great heights without climbing through the clouds.

◆　　　◆　　　◆

CHAPTER 1

Pros and Cons

Don't believe anything you hear . . .
and even less of what you see.

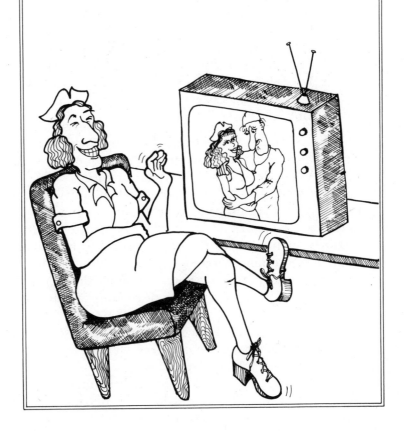

Fool me once, shame on you.
Fool me twice, shame on me.

How do a couple of sharp professionals like you and me get conned so easily and so often? Is it because we're too gullible, too naive, too nice, too trusting, too unsure of our own judgment or worth? *Yes!*

- We've been conned into believing that nurses are a nicety, not a necessity.
- We've been conned into accepting the responsibility of an airline pilot for the pay and prestige of a parking lot attendant.
- We've been conned into believing that nurses could be replaced by hordes of less expensive workers at the drop of a hat (or cap).

Employers have held this threat over our heads for years. Yet even when nurses were in critically short supply, we didn't call their bluff. Why? Because we're too flea brained.

Let me explain. I have it on good authority that when you first put fleas in a jar, they vigorously jump up and down banging their little heads on the lid. It hurts! Those determined little buggers quickly learn to adjust the height of their jumps. They continue to leap about coming within a hair's breadth of the lid.

After a couple of days you can remove the lid, and the fleas won't jump out of the jar. They continue to jump just short of where the lid was.

We nurses have a lot in common with those fleas. After years of low ceilings and painful encounters, we have learned to jump only so high. Even when the lid is removed, we don't jump out of the jar.

Sometimes I think the lid hasn't been removed at all, we've just been conned into thinking it has. On my more pessimistic days I suspect the tin lid has merely been replaced by one of transparent plastic. Today we can see new heights, but we can't reach them.

From all the talk about liberation, equality, and professionalism, you'd think we could easily escape the jar. But when we jump higher, we still bump our heads. We still hurt.

Actually, very little has changed. For example, women still account for 99 percent of all secretaries and 1 percent of all plumbers. The gap between men's and women's wages has not decreased one red cent. (Well, maybe *one* cent.) Women are still the ones with dishpan hands. And nurses are still "just nurses" and not the full partners in the health care system that we have longed to be.

- We've been conned into believing that politics is a nasty business that is better left in the hands of men.

Women comprise only 2 percent of the Senate and 5 percent of the Congress. Talk about taxation without representation! It must be time for another tea party.

- We've been conned into believing that money is not the most powerful substance on this planet.

When I hear women denying their need for monetary reward, I am reminded of cognitive dissonance theory. That theory says that when your beliefs and your experience are at odds, you feel pain. Brain pain. Your mind seeks resolution.

If you can't change your experience, you alter your beliefs so there is less disparity. If you find you don't have much money, you simply tell yourself that you don't need much money. Since women know they can't earn nearly as much as men, they deny money's importance. Then they expend great effort searching for another means to validate their worth in a society that sees them as "worth less."

Seeking to avoid pain, we lower our expectations. The lower your expectations, the less likely you are to be disappointed. Unfortunately, if you expect to be poor, you will be. If you expect to be mistreated, you will be. You'll be poor and mistreated, but you won't be disappointed because you got what you expected.

To thrive, you have to have high expectations. If you set your sights on mole hills, you will never conquer mountains. *Moral: think mountains.*

- We've been conned into believing it's more important to be liked than respected.

A man who works with his hands is a laborer.
A man who works with his hands and his head is a craftsman.
A man who works with his hands, head, and heart is an artist.
And a woman who works with her hands and her heart is a nurse.

Give St. Francis credit for the first three lines. The last line is to no one's credit. Unfortunately, we've been conned into believing that nurses don't need heads, just good hands and big hearts.

While screening applicants for admission to nursing school, I was surprised and appalled by the low quality of many applicants. They couldn't read, "right," add, or subtract. I hesitated to even suggest they seek employment as beauticians or manicurists because I didn't think most of them should be allowed to handle sharp objects. Yet they were told by friends, relatives, and *high school counselors* that they would make good nurses.

- We've been conned into believing nursing is a duty, not a career.

Recalling a bit of her own ancient history, an older nurse wrote,

> I was called into scrub around midnight. At the time we were paid $3 a call whether it was for 1 hour or all night. When I grumbled, the surgeon chastised me, saying I should be "happy to serve."
>
> Naturally he was making several hundred dollars to my measly three. I told him that when I was paid as well as he was, I would be "happy to serve." Happy? I'd be hysterically happy!

- We've been conned into believing that hard work, like virtue, is its own reward.

> I wish I would have been more assertive when I recently got a new job. As my boss (a man, of course) and I were discussing my salary, it actually came down to being slightly less than my present salary. I made a statement to him, "That's OK. I don't want this job only for the money," and I accepted the job with an actual cut in pay!! Ouch! A promotion?

This paragraph from *The Managerial Woman* describes how differently men and women approach work and careers:

> Women see a career as personal growth, as self-fulfillment, as satisfaction, as making a contribution to others, as doing what one wants to do. While men indubitably want these things too, when they visualize a career they see it as a series of jobs, a progression of jobs, as a path leading upward with recognition and reward implied. In all the seminars we have taught we have never once seen a

woman refer to recognition or reward as part of her career definition.*

When a new hospice was being organized, the community sponsoring it assumed they could get a master's-prepared nurse to voluntarily direct it. They were told by nurse advisors that was utterly ridiculous. After all, there was an acute shortage of nurses, and those with advanced degrees were particularly scarce. Evidently their prayers were answered because they found one.

For a full year that nurse directed the hospice on a part-time basis under the supervision of a chaplain. Finally, she rebelled. Her "part-time" involvement consistently topped 40 hours a week. The salaried chaplain's "supervision" consisted of a once-a-week "How ya doin'?"

The last straw came at a banquet when she found herself handing out awards to volunteers. Her anger bubbled to the surface as she admitted to herself that she had indeed been taken. For all her work she was not even getting a token award.

The volunteers never dreamed that such a highly professional person was going without a salary. The salaried people—chaplains and counselors—who worked alongside her never offered any appreciation or praise for her efforts.

After months of subservient service, she demanded the directorship be removed from the chaplain's supervision. The director would only be accountable to the board. She also demanded the position be made full-time and carry a respectable salary.

That was 2 years ago. Today the hospice is a highly successful operation. She continues to give splendid direction, but she is directing as a professional, not as a volunteer.

Would she do it again? Probably. The need was so great and the patients' gratitude so rewarding, almost any nurse would have trouble resisting. I would. I'll bet you would too.

Unfortunately, our profession will not thrive as long as we are more duty bound than career bound. We will not be taken seriously by other professions until we lay claim to the reward and recognition that should accompany our hard work.

---

*Hennig, Margaret, and Jardim, Anne: The managerial woman, New York, 1977, Doubleday & Co., Inc., p. 33.

◆ We've been conned into believing the doctor is always right.

Hospital rules
1. The doctor is always right.
2. If the doctor is wrong, see rule 1.

One doctor rants and raves about "poor nursing care" on our unit in front of patients, visitors, and nurses, then storms off. I am left standing speechless by this unexpected attack and angry that I didn't "do something."

We have been conned into accepting abuse because, like battered wives, we think we have done something to provoke it. We think it must be our fault. Horsefeathers! The man's a jerk. Being a physician merely makes him a "professional" jerk.

It's not a matter of the nurse being too sensitive or the doctor being too insensitive. There's a lot more at stake here than rudeness or hurt feelings.

The doctor has cast aspersions on the quality of care being offered by those nurses, on that unit, and in that hospital. Being a physician, his words carry a lot of weight. The damage he is doing is impossible to calculate, but it is considerable. Situations like this start visions of malpractice suits dancing in my head.

Can you for one moment imagine the tables turned? Can you imagine a nurse deriding a physician in front of patients, visitors, and other doctors?

"Geez, what a quack! I wouldn't let you operate on my dog! Where'd you buy your diploma anyway? Don't you ever botch things up like this again, or I'll have you thrown off my unit!"

You can bet those would be the last words ever uttered by that nurse. At least, her last words as an employed nurse.

A patient (demanding, manipulative, wealthy) complained to her doctor that the nurses had been telling her what she was and was not to do! (This is a cardiac rehabilitation unit where we monitor a patient's response to gradually increasing activity.)

The doctor, upon hearing her complaint, stormed into the station demanding that "one of the girls" explain what happened. Meek little me who always wants to smooth things out agreed to go into the patient's room with him to talk this out.

The doctor and I returned to the room. His statement to the patient was, "This one will apologize for all of the nurses. Now don't pay any attention to the nurses. They don't know what they're talking about. You just listen to me."

I was so upset I couldn't speak. Later, when I tried to talk to the physician about what had happened, he replied, "Well, that's how you have to handle a woman like that."

This doctor has been conned into believing that women—nurses and patients—have to be "handled."

♦ We've been conned into believing there is a health care team.

The dictionary defines teamwork as "work done by several associates with each doing a part but all subordinating personal prominence to the efficiency of the whole."

Nurses can easily set aside personal prominence. We have so little, it's not much of a sacrifice. Doctors, on the other hand, enjoy a great deal of personal prominence. To set theirs aside is a major sacrifice.

Every day, health care professionals attired in various uniforms traipse out onto the playing field. Since we don't practice together, we are never sure of just what the game plan is. We never know what our teammates are going to do next.

Some hog the ball. Others insist on running toward opposing goals. No one seems to know the score. Watching doctors and nurses play, you'd hardly know we were on the same side.

It was brought to the attention of the staff nurses that the doctors felt the nurses weren't treating them as professionals and were being unprofessional in their conduct. I suggested that a meeting be held with a panel of doctors and a panel of nurses to air our problems. The idea was put down by the medical staff and dropped.

What was the purpose of this skirmish? Certainly it served no useful purpose. Quite the contrary.

Here is a skirmish where doctors and nurses worked together to score a touchdown:

We were having problems with both doctors and nurses when it came to accurately recording intakes and outputs. The day shift blamed the night shift for errors. The night shift blamed the evening shift. Talking about the importance of I & Os did little or no good.

The doctors were irate. They griped constantly. They wrote on the doctor's orders in big, bold, black letters: **DO I & O AND RECORD.** They "bad mouthed" the nurses in their weekly medical meetings. The problem continued.

Our solution? We created a task force composed of three doctors and three nurses (one from each unit in our department) to meet, discuss the problem, and propose solutions.

Group communication was open and heated. Each person aired his or her feelings. Immediately there was a change for the better. After 6 months, the situation had improved so dramatically that the medical staff highly commended the nurses for their effort.

The task force has remained operational. Problem solving has been an ongoing process. The group deals with any problem, large or small. There are no more temper tantrums. The doctors and nurses have become real partners in patient care, and everyone is much happier.

Finding a multidisciplinary team that is alive, well, and fully functioning is a rare but exhilarating experience. Such teams are founded on intense mutual respect. Often all members are on a first-name basis. Information flows freely. Decision making is shared. Members take turns being "captain" based on patient needs at the time.

Finding a winning health care team is possible but not probable.

- We've been conned into believing that we are not only responsible for everyone's health and well-being, we are responsible for their happiness too.
- We've been conned into believing that health care is a right. Furthermore, we've been conned into believing it is our responsibility to provide that care cheaply, abundantly, and eternally.

At a conference on geriatric nursing, a clinician told of a dilemma posed by a cantankerous 85-year-old woman. The woman had a history of COPD, right CVA with left hemiparesis, multiple MIs with CHF, and renal failure. As if this weren't enough, she was also an insulin-dependent diabetic with a seizure disorder.

As each medical crisis arose, she was rushed from the nursing home to the hospital. There they patched her up. As soon as she stabilized, they shuttled her back to the nursing home.

Once back at the nursing home, she indulged in all her former vices that would precipitate the need for emergency care again . . .

and soon! She smoked incessantly, sometimes polishing off three packs a day. She ate only what she liked. She had an insatiable craving for salty foods and sweets. She was also overly fond of alcohol.

The health care team began to tire of building her up only to have her tear herself down again. She had them trapped in a vicious circle. They knew they couldn't win, but their code of ethics made it impossible for them to walk away from the game.

She died leaving over $150,000 in unpaid hospital bills. Everyone agreed the money was less important than the huge amount of professional time, talent, and energy she had consumed.

Money, time, energy—once spent they cannot be recaptured to invest in another person. Accepting the fact that these precious resources are *limited* is the first step in allocating them wisely. One way to conserve is to stop trying to save people who don't want to be saved.

Out of necessity the pendulum is swinging. Although once viewed as a right, health is being seen as a responsibility. Each individual's responsibility.

- We've been conned into believing . . .

  Nice nurses don't ———————————————————————.

  Good nurses do ———————————————————————.

(Fill in the blanks yourself.)

- We've been conned into believing that it is more important to correct our weaknesses than to capitalize on our strengths. That's why we are always apologizing and homogenizing.

  When I was being interviewed for a job in mental health, I was asked about my "tendency to be aggressive or assertive." They asked me to promise "not to make waves."

- We've been conned into believing it doesn't matter who gets the credit as long as *we* know we've done a good job.

  I work in public health in an "unorganized county," which means we do not have a county health department.
  We had a food poisoning outbreak and did all the follow-up that was needed. We wrote the reports and did a "super job."
  The local town health officer called us in and asked for a copy of all our reports. Then he promptly told us he would make the report

to the state capitol for us because we did not have a physician on our staff and therefore were not "qualified" to answer any questions the state epidemiologist might ask.

Until we stand up and take credit for our good works, no one will know how much nurses actually do or are capable of doing. Anonymous nurses will never be considered essential. Nursing will not thrive until our contributions are acknowledged by the more respected professions, by the politically powerful who shape policy, and by the public at large.

Nurses can also be great con artists. Here's a wonderful example to share:

> We had just moved into a brand-new hospital building, and nothing seemed to be going right. The tube system failed, the diet carts were late, and the medications disappeared in the transport system.
>
> The nurses were overwhelmed. Patient census was high. Overtime was mounting. The doctors were irritable. Morale was in the pits.
>
> As head nurse, I was the target for disgruntled nurses, irate doctors, and unhappy patients. At the end of a particularly grueling day, a young surgeon approached. He proceeded to chew me up and spit me out.
>
> At first I was devastated. Then I was furious. Snatching a piece of paper from my desk, I printed "S— Doctor" in large letters at the top. I wrote the young surgeon's name on it and posted it on our bulletin board. In professional jargon, it was going to be my "excreta list."
>
> My staff nurses began to chuckle. One of the more artistic ones incorporated the "S" in a colorful Superman shield. Each day we added a physician's name to the list. There were so many who deserved the honor that choosing just one was difficult—but fun!
>
> The nurses went about doing their chores feeling very smug and smiling a lot. Morale went up 100 percent.
>
> As the days passed, I became a little concerned about our game. The doctors had obviously noticed the list. Some made a point of coming into the station to read it. At last one doctor cornered me and asked about it. "Oh," I chirped, "that's our SUPER DOCTOR LIST." He asked me how to get his name on the list, and I told him the nurses voted at the end of each day.
>
> From that day on doctors actually began competing with one another for the privilege of being on the list. They smiled, an-

swered questions politely, asked if there was anything they could do to help. They engaged nurses in consultations, invited them along when they had something interesting to do, shared information from articles they had just read, and offered to teach in-service sessions.

Overnight, the list did become the SUPER DOCTOR LIST. And our doctors really became super.

CHAPTER 2

Promises, Promises
. . . and Other Propaganda

Where do we go from here?

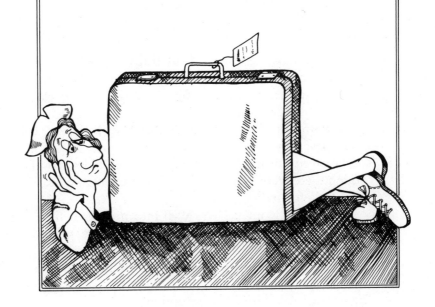

> *Whither thou goest, I will go.*
> *Whither thou lodgest, I will lodge.*
> *Thy people shall be my people*
> *And thy god, my god.*

$\mathbf{O}$h, my god, we're moving again.

Some nurses are frustrated because they can't stay in one community long enough to establish a career. Others are frustrated because they are unable to leave their community to pursue a career. Women who find themselves in such a quandary have been referred to as "tied stayers" and "tied movers." As a woman who is definitely "tied" to a man, I have experienced both.

When my husband and I were married back in 1966, we were both in graduate school. Since he was an aspiring physicist, I knew the places he would be able to work would be limited. We both thought it fortunate that I was a nurse and, therefore, *portable.* Nurses can get work anytime, anywhere. Promises, promises. . . .

With each move Gary's career advanced: a better position, a better salary, and better fringe benefits. As the "portable partner," I trailed along happily. I managed to find or create jobs that suited my fancy.

As our sons were born, I fitted my "career" around our family life. I was more interested in flexible schedules than fringe benefits. I never questioned the salary offered. Opportunities for advancement were never even discussed.

It wasn't until our last move that I really resented the whither-thou-goest clause in our marriage. I found myself exiled to the southeastern corner of Washington state. Sidelined. Derailed. Although there were "jobs" available, there were no "career" opportunities here for me.

Like most women I was well into my 30s before I grasped the real difference between jobs and careers. Jobs keep you busy. Careers build something of value.

After that last move, I began to recount my professional travels, reviewing my former jobs. Some were fun, some fascinating, some frustrating. All culminated in nothing.

While Gary was rewarded with each move, I was penalized. My salary, vacation time, pension fund, level of responsibility, and place on the totem pole were reduced to ground zero. In each new community I had to start from scratch. I had to *prove* myself over and over again.

When I arrived in the never-green part of the Evergreen State, something snapped. I just didn't want to start all over again. Besides, we were only going to be here for 2 years. That was 6 years ago.

Sometimes I feel like a helium balloon tied to an anchor. My husband provides a lot of security and stability. My problem is that I don't carry enough weight to budge him. When I shared this feeling with a friend, she suggested I just get a longer string. Now you know why I am so high strung.

When my husband and I entered our respective professions, our salaries were nearly equal. In our early years we used to talk about my finding the next job and his taking time off for other things. Today that possibility is highly implausible. It would be economically devastating for our family to try to live on my earnings.

Sadly, I've learned that jobs for nurses are plentiful but nursing careers are few and far between. "Go into nursing," I was counseled. "It's a good profession to fall back on." I guess they thought I would keep my nursing diploma in a box on the wall labeled "In case of emergency, break glass."

Education for a woman is often considered more like an insurance policy than preparation for a serious career. Our first duty is to be wives and mothers. If something should happen to our husbands (heaven forbid!), we would have a meager but respectable means of making a living.

It's comforting to know I have a profession to fall back on. There are millions of "fallen" women out there who don't have any sort of marketable job skills to back them up. Millions who believed those promises of perpetual care so completely that they never learned how to take care of themselves.

Even though statistics show almost every woman will be forced to go it alone at some point in her life, we refuse to believe it. We fail to prepare ourselves emotionally, intellectually, politically, or financially.

Statistically speaking, you have better than a 40 percent chance of being divorced. Yet you have only a 14 percent chance of being awarded alimony and only a 60 percent chance of being awarded child support (Census Bureau survey 1978). Actually, that survey found only 10 percent ever received any alimony. Of the women who were supposed to receive child support, half received the full amount, one fourth received partial payment, and one fourth received nothing at all. In 1984 the average child-support payment was only $40 per week.

Statistically speaking, you also have a *90 percent* chance of being widowed. So even if you are as lucky as I was to find a high-fidelity husband who promises you undying love, you can scratch the "undying" part. Try as we will, we just can't keep the little buggers alive.

Women still outlive men by an average of over 7 years. The average age of widowhood is 56. By age 65 half of all women are widowed. The Older Women's League (OWL) reports that only two of every ten women receive any pension based on their own or their husband's earnings. If you don't want to wind up rummaging through trash cans for your next meal, you'd better plan ahead.

For instance, if you want to decrease or eliminate widowhood, you should marry a man 8 or 10 years your junior. Women in their 20s find that advice obscene, in their 30s laughable, in their 40s conceivable, in their 50s preferable, and in their 60s necessary.

Women have been threatening that entering the work place shoulder-to-shoulder with men will take years off their lives. Threat? Sounds more like a promise to me. If it ever comes down to a choice between quantity and quality of life, I'd prefer to go for quality. I'd rather lop 10 years off my life than spend them alone, poor, cold, sick, or hungry. Besides, I don't believe that poppycock.

Originally I thought my marginal salaries and minimal advancement opportunities were correlated with my disconnected work history. On closer examination I discovered that staying in one community and working for one institution would have made no difference. (It wasn't Gary's fault after all!)

As a woman and a nurse, I would have reached the peak of my earning potential within 5 to 7 years. Then as "cost-of-living" raises failed to keep pace with the actual cost of living, my buying power would have steadily eroded.

In 1979 women aged 45 to 54 who worked full time had an average annual income of $10,935. That's only about 20 percent more than women aged 22 to 44 who averaged $8,902. In contrast, male workers over 45 averaged $20,465 or double what the younger male group averaged ($10,410).

So you see, I haven't lost much by being portable. I am just paying the heavy financial penalties this planet imposes on female occupants.

This spring I was unexpectedly offered an excellent position in a city I love. The salary was very respectable—for a nurse. Unfortunately, it was less than half my husband's salary. The "impractical" nurse in me longed to take the position. The "practical" nurse in me knew better.

I had just spent a year and a half setting up a school of nursing 300 miles from my home. The opportunity had been so unique that although I found it difficult to accept the position, I found it impossible to decline.

Gary backed me to the hilt. For the first time since our marriage I lived alone while Gary and the boys managed by themselves. Whenever possible I made a mad dash for home. Then our sons (Eric, 15, and Ryan, 11) elected to spend the school year with me. It was Gary's turn to live alone. It was his turn to make the long drive to be with his family.

Our phone bills were astronomical. After 18 months our tires and patience were wearing thin. Although our marriage was as strong as ever, we found long-distance parenting extremely difficult. It was with a strange mixture of grief and relief that I polished off the project and hired my replacement.

What an adventure! Would I do it again? Yes. Or so I thought until the phone rang and I was offered a wonderfully attractive position *only* 200 miles from home. That's when I realized I had not fully recovered. This time I declined. I had other promises to keep.

Women have been criticized for their high turnover rates, yet when consideration is given to the types of jobs that foster high turnover—low-paying, dead-end jobs with little opportunity for advancement, marginal economic rewards, and minimal respect—the turnover rate is the same for men and women.

It *appears* women have higher turnover rates because we have nearly cornered the market on crummy jobs. And we're so cheap! Take a man and a woman in the same crummy job. Give them a *1 percent* increase in salary, and she is three times less likely to quit than the man. Women continue to take jobs that no self-respecting man would touch. That's because women are not self-respecting.

We work hopefully ever after. Fairy tales taught us that a miserable life was mandatory if we wanted to marry a prince. They promised us that no matter how poor, tired, hungry, overworked, or underloved a woman was, Prince Charming was only a kiss away.

If you look closely at yourself, you might see a trace of Little Red Riding Hood, Mother Hubbard, Sleeping Beauty, Cinderella, Snow White, or other fairy tale characters.

Take *Little Red Riding Hood.* Are you the kind of nurse who gets in trouble because you fail to follow directions or take foolish shortcuts? Are you so nearsighted that you can't see danger (or opportunity) looming right before your eyes? Are you fair game for wolves?

Perhaps you're more like *Mother Hubbard.* Maybe you're the kind of nurse who not only gives till it hurts, you give till it's gone. You look after everyone's needs but your own. You're uncomfortable when people offer you compliments, assistance, advice, goods, or services. Even when your cupboard is bare, you go through the motions of giving even though it is just an empty gesture.

If you find the men you work for or live with come up short, you have a lot in common with *Snow White.* Helping little people is fine, but you don't want to work for one or marry one. Snow White is cheerful, hardworking, and industrious but also naive, compliant, and too trusting of the wrong people.

Sleeping Beauty closes her eyes to anything unpleasant or strenuous. She dreams of a cottage, adoring husband, and adorable children.

Rudely awakened by divorce, death, or the natural displacement that occurs as children mature and move away, a Sleeping Beauty often finds herself in dire straights—economically and emotionally. She dozed off when she should have been paying attention to insurance, investments, pension plans, personal development, and marketable job skills.

Like Sleeping Beauty many nurses are dreamers. That's one of the reasons why our profession has not matured. There are several other reasons why nursing remains essentially a young woman's profession. First, it is strenuous: physically, emotionally, and intellectually. Second, the long hours and irregular schedules make it more suited to one who is personally unencumbered. Third, it requires exorbitant amounts of idealism and optimism. Fourth, the salary and advancement opportunities can only satisfy naive or immature professionals.

Many nurses prefer to keep their eyes closed, but some of us are quite alert. We are waking to find nurses cannot always get a job anytime, anywhere. Seeing that promise broken for the first time makes many nurses feel betrayed. We were childish to believe nursing was a forever profession.

We were foolish to think unused knowledge and skills wouldn't decay. We were foolish to think women who walked (or ran) away from nursing years ago could step back in as if nothing has changed. We now realize that no one can fall back on nursing. You have to run to keep up.

Finally we're waking up, and we're growing up. After years of being politically unconscious, all Sleeping Beauties are showing signs of arousal. In the 1980 national election women voted at the same percentage rate as men for the first time in history. Up until then women had always lagged so far behind men in voting numbers that pollsters never bothered to include us in their surveys.

Well, we're awake, and we don't like what we see. We are just catching on to what politicians mean when they say, "Women and children first." They mean to throw us over the side of the economic lifeboat right along with the elderly and the infirm. Instead of closing our eyes and waiting for those same men to rescue us, we are voting in record numbers. From now on you can bet women will be polled.

There is another beauty in the Fairy Tale Hall of Fame: *Beauty and the Beast.* In this scenario men are beasts, and women are duty bound to save them.

When I was a student nurse on clinical rotation in Chicago, a psychologist speaking to our class said, "Nurses marry weak, dependent men." I was flabbergasted. By the time I got to the dorm, I was furious. How dare she say something like that!

As I grew calmer I began thinking about the kind of men I was attracted to—*losers.* There is something in me that responds deeply to need in others. I am drawn to people with handicaps, terminal illnesses, and quick but neurotic minds. I am a rescuer. Most nurses are rescuers.

The outspoken director of an alcoholic treatment center was discussing the types of people who make the best counselors. When nurses were mentioned, she blurted out, "Nurses? They're the worst! They always want to kiss everything and make it better."

Nurses work at salvaging human wreckage. Unfortunately, too many of us take our work home with us. We've been brainwashed to believe the love of a good woman can cure anything. We've been duped into believing that it is not only our duty to care for those less fortunate or able than ourselves, it is our duty to marry them! No wonder so few of us live happily ever after.

Once upon a time if you finished all your household chores, you got to go to the ball. If today's *Cinderella* gets all her household chores done, she gets to go to a job.

The 1980 United Nations Report on the Status of Women said that women do 66 percent of the world's work. I was not surprised. Most women I know put in 8 hours on the job and then rush home to another full-time shift as homemaker.

What astounded me in that UN report was the fact that for all our work, *women receive less than 10 percent of the world's income and own less than 1 percent of the world's property.* Put another way, men receive 90 percent of the world's income and own 99 percent of the world's property. They did get the gold mine. We did get the shaft.

Women are still waiting in the ashes hoping for a fairy god-mother to come along. We still believe it is magic, not money, that will transform our lives.

In her excellent book, *The Cinderella Complex,*★ Colette Dowling talks about women's yearnings for dependence. She feels the chief force holding women down is their deep-seated wish to be taken care of by others.

Two of the phrases in her book that particularly stuck with me are "collapse of ambition" and "dwindling into a wife." They are so descriptive of what happens to me and many other nurses.

For example, a group of highly credentialed coronary care nurses were complaining about being abused. They were exhausted from working double shifts, carrying heavy patient loads, and being forced to forego days off and cancel vacations.

Seeing their plight, a nurse administrator advised them to do what physicians had done long ago. She suggested they form a cor-poration and then sell their services back to the institution under their own terms. Immediately she witnessed what could only be described as a depressing "collapse of ambition" as every one of them "dwin-dled" into a nurse right before her eyes.

Those coronary care nurses could not see the opportunity pre-

---

★Dowling, Colette: The Cinderella complex: women's hidden fear of independence, New York, 1981, Summit Books.

sented by incorporating. They only saw the risk and danger. The thought terrified them.

Watching their courage and confidence evaporate, the nurse administrator felt very sad. Her hopes for nursing's eventual autonomy also dwindled. If highly educated, experienced, and talented nurses fled from autonomy, she doubted the rest of us garden-variety nurses could be expected to strive for it.

The Cinderella Complex offers a compelling explanation for nursing's failure to successfully extricate itself from domination by more powerful professions. Nursing is a woman's profession. Women long for dependence.

Fairy tale women can be excused for being "Grimm." They're ancient history. Let's update our make-believe world a bit.

I love watching old movies on TV, but many of the lines uttered by my favorite leading men make me cringe. Lines like, "Women and dogs—the more you beat them, the better they are" and "There are two kinds of women: mothers and the other kind."

Career women are not portrayed kindly, and no matter how successful they are, as soon as the male lead whistles, they drop everything and retire to the suburbs. When a classy woman is being courted by two men, she invariably chooses the poorer, weaker one rather than the richer, stronger, more successful one. That's romance? That's stupid!

Every day we see Buddy Hackett-dumpling-type men stroll off into the sunset with statuesque blondes. Just once I would like to see a plump, bespectacled woman (with a great personality) walk off with a Cary Grant look-alike. But that will never happen. Why? Because nobody would believe it.

In vintage movies and television series, men used to have all the action, fun, and adventure. Today men still have all the action, fun, and adventure.

Richard Levinson of Emory University studied Saturday morning television from 1969 to 1973 and from 1974 to 1978. During that time he found females accounted for only 25 percent of the characters in children's programing. What those few women lacked in quantity, they also lacked in quality. He found women generally relegated to negative, stereotypical roles and portrayed as weak, passive, less interesting, and less active than men.

Reviewing award-winning children's books over the same time period, he noted an increase in female characters from 18 percent in

1969 to 34 percent by 1978. Although the percentage of female characters almost doubled, males still comprised 82 percent of the *main* characters. In 1978 Levinson found male characters portrayed in 95 different occupational roles compared with a paltry 19 for women.

And we were promised things were changing.

No wonder preschool boys were upset when asked, "If you were a girl, what would you like to be when you grow up?" They couldn't think of anything worse than being a girl. "Yuck!" When preschool girls were asked, "If you were a boy, what would you like to be when you grow up?", they responded quickly and positively with dozens of different answers.

Women fare poorly on television. How do nurses fare? The made-for-television nurse had her prime time in the 1960s. An hour-long dramatic series, *The Nurses,* aired on CBS from 1962 to 1965. The series conveyed a highly positive image of the nursing profession, allowing nurses to be both compassionate and assertive, caring and intelligent, warm and decisive. The series also explored every facet and variety of nursing practice.

In the 1970s more nurses popped up on television shows than ever before. Unfortunately, they were more decorative than useful. They interacted with doctors instead of patients.

In the 1980s nurses are primarily "extras" and rarely main characters. They are still mostly decorative. They often serve as the butt of practical jokes. They are also used as sponges to absorb verbal barrages from irate doctors. After all, someone has to listen to those self-righteous tirades writers love to pen for the script's doctor.

Forty or fifty years ago movie scripts made nurses saints. Today nurses are more likely to be cast as sluts or sinister characters bent on hurting instead of helping.

It's been said that art imitates life. If that's true, the lives of most women and nurses could be summed up in one word: boring.

Advertisements make a lot of promises. I clipped a large ad for a Dale Carnegie Course out of the newspaper. The heading read, "New Year's Resolution for 1984: TAKE ACTION!" Below the heading were pictures of two of their graduates. One was a close-up of an absolutely gorgeous young woman identified as Bonnie Montgomery. Under her picture it says, "I know how to face and accept rejection."

Beside her picture is one of a young man, Bill Walkiewicz. He is shown at his desk examining papers. On the wall behind him is an award plaque. The camera has literally given him a better background than Bonnie. In fact, Bonnie has no background at all. Under his picture it says, "I learned how to set goals and make a plan to accomplish those goals."

Only a woman would see accepting rejection as a major accomplishment. Only a woman would want to be a "successful" failure.

Women who give up everything for love and men who give up everything for work eventually learn to their dismay that they based their lives on false promises. To thrive, a life must be built equally on both love and work.

And that's the truth. I promise.

CHAPTER 3

Procreation

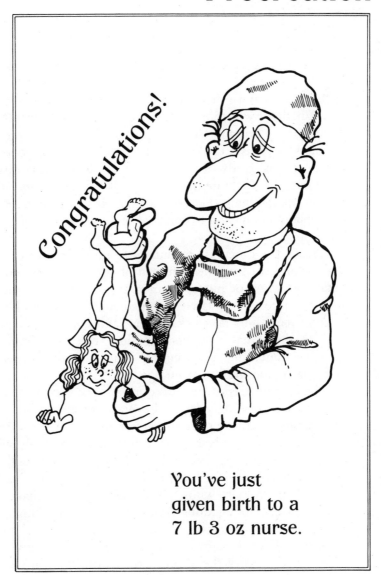

You've just
given birth to a
7 lb 3 oz nurse.

Are nurses born or made?

Whether by birthing or by manufacturing, it takes 2 to 5 years of hard labor to bring forth a new registered nurse. The creation process requires one basic raw material: people. Finding people willing to undertake the study of nursing may be increasingly difficult.

First, the birthrate has declined. There are simply fewer young people approaching that critical first-career decision. All trades and professions are having to compete more vigorously for their share of the young.

Second, women are beginning to move into career fields previously dominated by men. Instead of choosing between being a secretary, teacher, or nurse, women are choosing to study computer science, accounting, law, and medicine. They are becoming mechanics, coal miners, truck drivers, and construction workers. Although the actual numbers adopting such "nonfeminine" careers remains minuscule, the trend is being carefully observed, highly publicized, and ideally encouraged.

These two trends help account for the fact that enrollment in schools of nursing has declined every year since 1978.

Because there are not enough young people to go around, attention is being focused on people in their 30s and 40s who are contemplating a midlife career change. Many men, disillusioned with their present jobs, are looking for more satisfying career alternatives. Many women, whose family responsibilities have decreased or whose financial obligations have increased, are looking at entering or reentering the job market.

The bulk of these people are not as naive as they were at age 18. They cannot afford the altruism of youth. They are asking serious questions about salaries, working conditions, fringe benefits, and opportunities for advancement. Can nursing attract and hold their interest?

Even young people appear to be less naive and altruistic than they once were. Each year the American Council on Education and the University of California at Los Angeles survey college freshmen. In their report, "The American Freshman: National Norms for Fall 1982," they say freshmen are more materialistic and show less social concern than in past years.

Consistent with a trend that began in the mid 1970s, the freshmen place *less* importance on cleaning up the environment, helping people in difficulty, promoting racial understanding, developing a meaningful philosophy, or giving preferential treatment to the disadvantaged.

Record numbers of freshmen are moving toward the better-paying professions of business, engineering, and computer programing. Most say they are in college to "make more money." Almost 70 percent of the freshmen said that being "very well off financially" was an essential objective.

One nurse recruiter tells of speaking at a high school career day program. After explaining the various nursing education plans available, the licensure requirements, and some of the legal-ethical responsibilities of nurses, she was asked candidly about nurses' salaries. When she told them the current salary range, one obviously disappointed student replied, "That doesn't seem like much money for all you have to go through to be a nurse."

Although the recruiter quickly assured the group that nurses' salaries are getting better, she said silently to herself, "If you think the salaries are bad, wait until you get a load of the working conditions." Selling nursing is getting more difficult all the time.

The problems nurses encounter are a microcosm of the problems women encounter. Our profession is still 97 percent female. Facing the truth about life as a nurse may be as painful as facing the truth about life as a woman. Painful but necessary for survival.

While attending meetings of the American Association for the Advancement of Science (San Francisco, 1979), I happened upon a session concerning women and birth order. The speaker reported polls showing 80 percent of American couples, given a choice, would elect to have a male child first. She was concerned because there is evidence that firstborn children are likely to have higher IQs, better verbal skills, and a tendency to be high achievers.

As I listened, I began thinking about the field day science fiction writers could have with this piece of information. Imagine a future in which there are no firstborn females. Certainly technology enabling us to select the sex of our unborn children is imminent. Perhaps it is already available. . . .

My momentary daydream was interrupted when the speaker turned to the large, predominantly female audience and asked all the firstborn people in the room to raise their hands. A gasp went up as fully 95 percent of us, myself included, raised our hands. She simply nodded and said, "It happens every time."

As the session concluded, she left us with a haunting question: "Why don't women want to reproduce themselves?" That fascinating and frightening question still surfaces frequently in my mind.

Eventually her question coupled with the escalating nurse shortage triggered another question in my mind: "Do nurses want to reproduce themselves?"

While conducting workshops across the United States and Canada, I began looking for the answer. I asked hundreds of nurses to write their responses to the following:

"Your daughter (son) is about to graduate from high school. Give her (him) three convincing reasons why she (he) should consider becoming a nurse."

1. _____

2. _____

3. _____

Take a moment to fill in your own responses.

If you have difficulty coming up with three convincing reasons why *any* young person should consider a career in nursing, especially one as important as your own son or daughter, you are not alone.

After gathering the responses, I usually ask workshop participants how difficult it was to come up with three reasons. When given a scale from one to ten with ten being the most difficult, someone frequently chirps, "an eleven!" The majority agree that the task was difficult. For many it was impossible.

"I can't—I told both of my daughters not to go into nursing."
"Encourage my son or daughter to go into nursing? *Never!*"
"I really don't think I could give her three good reasons to become a nurse—in fact, I don't think I could give her *one!*"

One respondent wrote, "I spent 3 years convincing my daughter that there were other career fields offering her more respect, more pay, more personal rewards, and less physical exhaustion."

Another listed three convincing reasons *not* to consider nursing:

1. Society still thinks nurses are the brainless handmaidens of the world.
2. Nursing education programs are worse than Marine boot camp.
3. It is impossible to support a family on a nurse's salary.

With friends like these nursing doesn't need any enemies. The time has come to take a good look at ourselves and our colleagues. Are we walking advertisements for the nursing profession, or are we walking warnings discouraging people from considering nursing as a career?

Take your own poll. Ask the nurses on your unit, in your hospital, or at your nurses' association meeting to write down three convincing reasons for entering the nursing profession. You will easily identify nurses who are burned up, burned out, or still brimming with enthusiasm. Their responses make an excellent springboard for discussions of what's right and what's wrong with our profession. We urgently need to right the wrongs, so nursing can remain a viable career choice.

What's right with nursing? Consistently the *number one* reason given to encourage a son or daughter to consider a career in nursing is: "You can always get a job." In fact, "You can always get a job anywhere in the world."

The second most frequently given reason is that the profession is "personally rewarding." A close third is a host of humanitarian reasons centered around "helping others."

Some other "convincing" reasons include:

The ever-popular "meet-and-marry-a-doctor."
"Challenging! Nursing pushes me to my limits."
"It's good training for motherhood."
"You don't need a large wardrobe to work."
"It's a good profession to fall back on—sort of like Social Security (and just as solvent?)."
"Lots of variety."
"You never have to worry about being in a high tax bracket."

If you are an optimist or an opportunist, you might see this as an excellent time to enter a floundering profession.

"The *future* in nursing looks good!"
"You can only move *up!*"

Those viewing nursing most favorably fall into two categories: unemployed nurses and nurses who hold health care jobs outside of hospitals. Many view nursing as an excellent stepping stone to more flexible, creative, autonomous jobs inside and outside the health care system.

Lately there is every evidence that nursing may be losing its foremost point of appeal—"You can always get a job." If the economic recession/depression of the early 1980s does nothing else, it has managed to ease, if not virtually eliminate, the nurse shortage. Part-time nurses began asking to work full-time as their husbands' jobs were threatened or lost. Nurses who hadn't darkened the door of a hospital in years suddenly enrolled in refresher courses and signed on to work. Within months the nurse shortage became a nurse surplus.

Educators and recruiters may view this turn of events as either a problem or an opportunity, but for the first time in years the pressure is off. As long as the demand for nurses exceeded the supply, the profession was pressured to step up the manufacturing process. The advent of associate degree nursing programs was one result. No matter how many new nurses graduated each year, institutions seemed to gobble them up and cry out for more. In our haste to manufacture the right quantity, some fear we have sacrificed our commitment to quality.

The idea of making the baccalaureate degree the entry level into professional practice is an idea whose time has come . . . and gone . . . and perhaps come again. During this respite when we are not driven to manufacture vast quantities of nurses, we have the opportunity to reevaluate and, if necessary, revamp nursing education.

Right now, to become a nurse you must successfully survive an educational process lasting anywhere from 2 to 5 years. The fact that it takes some people twice as long as others to become nurses causes conflict inside the profession and confusion outside the profession. Our indecisiveness is embarrassing.

Since we have never delineated exactly what services a nurse will provide, we must guess at what she needs to know to be equal to the task. And the "task" of nursing seems to encompass everything from providing the most elementary physical care to performing the most sophisticated research.

Attempting to define nursing, one man wrote, "Nursing is what nurses do. And nurses *do everything!*" The expectation that a nurse must be a "jack-of-all-trades and master of 'some' " is unrealistic. No wonder nurses are anxious. No wonder we are obsessed with education. How do you educate someone to "do everything"?

Ars longa, vita brevis.

Translation: "The life so short, the craft so long to learn."

Although encouraging a commitment to lifelong learning may be desirable, nurses seem to have an unhealthy compulsion to educate, reeducate, and continually educate. Perhaps our educational goal is so unclear we don't recognize it when we reach it.

Few students are adequately counseled about the strengths and limitations of the various nursing education programs available. Their choice is not determined by past performance, future potential, or long-range career goals. Most often it is determined by whichever program is quickest, cheapest, or closest to home.

For decades problems of educational mobility have plagued nursing. For a while the career ladder concept seemed promising. That concept is based on the assumption that a common information core exists, which can be built on at any future time. Logically, with additional education and experience, an able nurse's aide should be able to move up to the practical nurse level, and a practical nurse should be able to move up to the associate degree level and become a registered nurse.

This ladder works well through the associate degree level. At that point, halfway up the educational ladder, many nurses seem to be stuck. Those wishing to pursue their studies for a bachelor of science in nursing degree are essentially told they have to start at the bottom and make the whole climb again.

One very successful director of nursing (a diploma graduate) shared her difficulties when she tried to pursue a BSN degree. At the state university she was told her previous experience and education were worth a sum total of nine college credits. Angry and frustrated, she turned away from the school of nursing and is now completing her master's in business administration.

When a hospital diploma program and a private college merged to offer both a generic BSN program and an external degree BSN

31

program (one that would be offered off campus at different locations throughout the state), the response was overwhelming. Before the program officially opened, the college had received 14,000 requests for information, and 3500 nurses visited the campus personally.

In spring 1982 I was hired to set up an associate degree nursing program for a small community college in Oregon. While I was busily laying the foundation for the new program, the Oregon State Board of Nursing made a motion to require the baccalaureate degree for entry into professional practice by 1990. That motion caused an uproar.

Overnight two camps formed: those who supported associate degree nursing education and those who supported baccalaureate nursing education. In hopes of minimizing polarization, nurse educators quickly formed a special interest group consisting of the deans and directors of the state's various nursing programs.

Dialogue was spirited. If the ADN backers were guilty of trying to teach their students to *do* everything, then the BSN backers were guilty of trying to teach their students to *be* everything. Supporters of baccalaureate education campaigned for one level of nursing practice—professional. Supporters of associate degree education campaigned for two levels of nursing practice—technical and professional.

In one important area the ADN educators had a distinct advantage. They knew the limits of their graduates. Their scope of practice had already been carefully defined and published. Feeling the role, education, identification, licensure, and employment of the "technical" nurse were well established, they challenged the BSN educators to address the same issues for the "professional" nurse.

During these lively exchanges, the nurse educators discovered that they had more in common than any one of them had dared hope. All recognized this was not a "we-they" problem but an "us" problem. The group set about changing the problem into an opportunity. Resolution was no longer a dream but a goal.

At first glance those Board of Nursing motions appeared to have lit a fuse. Now it appears they actually lit a candle. Oregon may become a light to lead the way. Although early discussions picked at whether registered nurses *should* or *must* have baccalaureate degrees, later discussions focused on the real questions: who, what, when, where, why, how, and how much?

When college presidents, legislators, and others offered their muscle and advice, they were told this was an intraprofessional problem and the nurses would handle it. That's leadership.

The decision to support one or two levels of nursing education may not be as important as the fact that a decision is made and that nurses make it.

> So important is the timing of a decision in some situations that *any* resolution of a problem is better than none. It is easy to see that the best decision made too late is—well, too late. What is more difficult to accept is that a bad decision is often better than none.★

This is our profession. It is our right and responsibility to determine how future nurses will be created, licensed, and utilized. If we fail to make these decisions, they will be made for us.

★Mackenzie, R. Alec: The time trap: managing your way out, New York, 1972, AMACOM Book Division, pp. 113-114.

7

CHAPTER 4

Procuring and Keeping Nurses

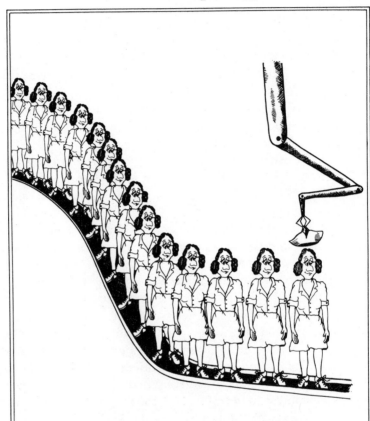

Factory-direct disposable nurses.

Wholesale price.

Interchangeable parts.

See our catalogue for details.

Let's talk about headhunters. Not the kind you find in the wilds of Borneo but the sophisticated kind. The ones who hunt top-notch professionals and outstanding executives. Corporations pay such headhunters handsome sums because they know the value of having the right person in the right job. They also know the cost of having the wrong person.

Unfortunately, when it comes to filling nursing vacancies, hospitals don't hunt heads, they hunt *herds!* Large, docile herds of nurses who will meander in, graze awhile, and then move on to greener pastures.

When it comes to nurses, hospitals have always been more interested in quantity than quality. That's because they can count better than they can think.

There are several reasons why hospitals don't engage in head-hunting. One is that nurses are not thought to need very good heads. They are literally hired hands. In fact, many who employ and manage nurses prefer nurses who are not very "head strong." Another reason is that head-hunting looks expensive. Hospitals are penny-wise and pound-foolish institutions. Third, luring an outstanding nurse away from her present employer by offering her more money is too radical an idea. It flies in the face of one of hospitaldom's oldest beliefs: nurses are interchangeable. Besides, if the herd got wind of it, they might stampede.

Traditionally hospitals have been content to make do with whatever nurses they had on hand. If they didn't happen to have enough on hand, they sat back and waited for some to wander in.

Until the new "stock" arrived, the old staff was prodded to work longer and harder: take on double shifts, forego days off, and increase patient loads. Under the strain many loyal, long-term nurse employees resigned.

The herd-management mentality persisted saying, "Well, that's just the way nurses are. They don't stay in any hospital very long. They are always looking for greener pastures." Even when the nurse shortage became critical, hospitals balked at making their own grasses greener.

The nurse shortage escalated. Soon even hospitals with religious affiliations didn't have a prayer when it came to acquiring the nurses they needed. Nurses were staying away from hospitals in droves. Desperation increased.

Hospitals tried to maintain their high standards for hiring nurses: "If it's walking, breathing, and licensed—hire it!" As the shortage wore on, they began settling for two out of three.

One vacationing nurse happened upon a lovely little community. She was so attracted to the spot that she called the hospital and the two nursing homes located there. All three tried to hire her over the phone, sight unseen!

Another nurse decided to go on a round of interviews just to see what else might be available in her city. During the first few moments of one interview she was asked if she had brought a uniform with her. At another institution she was asked if she could begin work that evening.

Clinging to the belief that it was more important to find new nurses than to hold their own, hospitals poured money into newspaper and journal advertisements. They took out bigger, better, and longer-running classified ads. One hospital laughingly became known as "Our Lady of the Perpetual Want Ad."

But nurses had become more astute at reading those ads. We knew that "competitive salaries" meant they paid the exact same salary as every other institution in the area. We knew "challenging positions" meant twice the work for the same salary. In short, the more elaborate the ad, the lower the salary and the heavier the work load.

Reluctantly hospitals began to relinquish another of their most cherished beliefs: nurses are disposable. Besides attracting new nurses, they realized the necessity of keeping their old ones. Resisting the obvious (raising salaries, increasing fringe benefits, and improving working conditions), they offered minor prizes, gimmicks, and gags: laundry service, free parking, all the coffee you could drink. Eventually those Cracker Jack prizes grew into cash bounties, new cars for night nurses, and trips to Hawaii.

(When they were just on the verge of having to offer something substantial, the entire economy of the United States collapsed and the shortage was solved . . . at least temporarily.)

At its peak the nurse shortage spawned countless theories, excuses, committees, commissions, and studies. The shortage also spawned a new position in many hospitals: nurse recruiter.

A nurse was singled out and given responsibility for solving the shortage at her particular hospital. Often she knew nothing of public relations, advertising, promotion, marketing, or personnel management. She was simply appointed and told to recruit.

At the height of the nurse shortage, I conducted a little experiment. I called all the hospitals in a large city and asked for their nurse recruiter. Using my sister's name and address, I told them I was moving into their city and wanted to find a job. I asked if there was anything special I should know about their hospital. I also requested any brochures or information they could send to help me learn about their facility.

I had created a thumbnail sketch of my experience, education, and interests so I would be consistent in what I shared with each recruiter. (That's not easy when you're a psych nurse who is trying to pass for a med-surg nurse.)

To my surprise—and relief—not one recruiter asked me any question about my personal or professional life. There was no attempt to engage me in conversation. They didn't ask me why I was moving to their city, what I had done professionally, how I had been educated, or what my interests were.

Few had any response to my question: "Is there anything special about your hospital? Is there something that sets it apart from the rest?" After some thought they might mention that they were a teaching-research facility or had a burn unit.

The only hospital that had no recruiter connected me immediately with an assistant director of nursing. She had a ready response to the above questions. Yes, they had something that set them apart. They had an all-RN staff and practiced primary care. Their turnover rate was only 5 percent a year, and they had a waiting list of nurses who wanted to come and work for them.

Isn't it fascinating that her information packet was the first to arrive? The nonrecruiter, who already had nurses waiting, sent me the requested information first class. Within 48 hours her brochures and application forms were in my hand.

Most of the mailings arrived within 7 days. There were a few stragglers, and one dawdling recruiter took 16 days to deliver any information.

The contents of the packets varied widely. Again, to my surprise, not one included a personal note or anything signed by the recruiter. There were no friendly overtures; no helpful hints to aid in my relocation; no maps or information on housing, schools, or neighborhoods. Nothing. Two recruiters, and I use the term loosely, sent application forms but absolutely no information about their hospitals, not even a picture postcard!

At a time when hospitals were reporting nurse turnover rates ranging from 40 to 100 percent, you can quickly see what an economic advantage the hospital with a 5 percent rate enjoyed. The cost of replacing nurses is staggering.

One way to estimate the cost of recruiting and orienting new nurses at your hospital is to use the American Management Association's formula. They multiply 500 times the hourly rate times the number of employees replaced. If a staff nurse makes $10 an hour, it would cost an estimated $5000 to replace her. If your institution employs 500 nurses and has a 40 percent turnover rate, they are replacing 200 nurses a year at an estimated cost of *1 million dollars!* It really pays to keep turnover rates down.

To gain insight into what attracts and holds nurses, I began using the following exercise:

"Your best friend from nursing school has just moved to your community. Give her three convincing reasons why she should come to work for your hospital (agency, clinic, institution)."

1. _____

2. _____

3. _____

When workshop groups are given this assignment, an alarming number of nurses are absolutely stumped. They have to think long and hard. Many barely manage one flimsy reason such as, "Well, we'd be together" or "We could car pool." Others have a single plea: "We need you desperately!"

Among workshop participants in large metropolitan areas, usually one hospital's employees are more vocal and more positive than others. When a particularly complimentary reason crops up like "Our nursing administration is dynamic and supportive," the audience is quick to ask, *"Where do you work!?"*

Public relations departments and personnel recruiters would find their present employees' responses to this simple exercise very enlightening. Every employee reflects both the image and substance of the institution. Each is either a walking warning or a walking advertisement for the facility.

Here are a few responses from employees who are walking-talking warnings:

> "I cannot think of *any* reason to work for my hospital. I'm beginning to wonder why *I* work for them. They offer absolutely nothing in the line of opportunity or real advancement."

> "Don't come to work here—very unstable—administration does not back you."

> "I work at 'Rufus Memorial.' Don't go there. Go to 'St. Ignats.'"

Here are one nurse's tongue-in-cheek reasons:

1. You can earn a tiny bit more money.
2. We can have a few laughs.
3. The doctors are extremely ignorant.

One nurse wrote *five* reasons:

1. Good pay
2. Good hours
3. Excellent opportunity for advancement
4. Really care about each employee
5. Bonuses paid for good attendance

That sounds great until you read her final note: "These are fictitious. I'm not employed. But if I could find an employer who would offer any of the above, I'd join the work force again!"

Perhaps the saddest comment, by virtue of its frequency, is: "Our hospital is no worse than any other." Think about it. Does your employer strive for excellence or do only the minimum to prevent slipping from a second-rate to a third-rate hospital?

When discussing reasons to work for an employer, the comments that draw the most audience interest are those related to supportive administrators who listen to suggestions and encourage creativity and autonomy.

Here are some of the reasons listed by employees who are happy to recommend their employers to their best friends:

"Supportive nursing administration"
"Good educational opportunities"
"Lots of intelligent, informed people"
"Friendly"
"Fair"
"Compassionate"
"Time and a half on weekends"
"Trend-setter"
"Computerized system"
"No rotating shifts"
"Superb patient care"
"Open to suggestions"
"Convenient location"
"Small-town atmosphere"
"Support for inventive ideas"
"Flexible schedules"
"Excellent salaries"
"Wonderful fringe benefits"
"Opportunities for personal growth"
"Challenging work"
"State-of-the-art equipment"
"Variety of positions"
"Newest and largest"
"Autonomy of practice"
"Job security"
"Encourages creativity"
"Allows ingenious people to produce"
"Great colleagues"
"Best hospital in town!"

Go back through that list and circle those descriptive phrases that apply to your hospital or employer. Jot down any other reasons to work for your employer here:

_____

_____

_____

If your list is a little thin, it's not unusual.

When it came to courting and keeping nurses, hospitals were notoriously cheap. Some even begrudged "spending" a thank-you on their nurses. Their no-deposit-no-return management style eventually proved their undoing. They refused to invest an extra nickel in their nurses, and their nurses stopped returning.

Turnover rates went from inconvenient to intolerable because turning over was the only way nurses could better their position. As long as a nurse stayed loyal to her employer, she was likely to be stuck on the wrong shift, on the wrong unit, and at a salary often lower than a newly hired nurse.

Lo and behold, nurses were not immune to overwork or impervious to insults and abuse. Loyal nurses began to demand loyalty from their employers. Nickels spent on recruitment had to be matched by nickels spent on retention efforts.

Hospitals began investing nickels in nurses. They spent one nickel on salaries, another on fringe benefits. They hired nurse recruiters and financed toll-free phone numbers, open houses, convention booths, fancy advertisements, and press parties.

They spent a few nickels on other inventive incentives to attract and hold their nurses including such things as free prescription drugs, free tax service, free coffee, cafeteria discounts, garden patches, memberships in recreation facilities at reduced prices, social events, jogging tracks, on-site child care, awards for good attendance, monetary bonuses for unused sick leave, and short-term cash advances on future earnings.

Seattle's Virginia Mason Hospital sponsors a Nurse Recognition Day. Peers vote for outstanding nurses. Winners are not only honored at a party, they are given a day off with pay.

Some of the best incentives to stay with an employer don't cost a cent. Courtesy and compliments are free. They are also highly contagious. Introduce them in your hospital, and they will spread like wildfire.

Too often compliments, like eulogies, are saved for the dearly departed. Until a nurse retires or resigns, no one bothers to tell her how much she is appreciated. Many insist if they had known how much they would be missed, they might not have quit.

When nurses are asked to share the last compliment they received in the workplace, the lack of examples is disheartening. When asked to share the last compliment they *gave* in the workplace, the silence is eloquent.

There are some notable exceptions like the nurse who found an envelope taped to her locker. In it was a letter from the director of nurses letting her know how much her efforts were appreciated. It contained specific examples of how she had helped patients, families, and colleagues and expressed the hope that she would remain on staff for a long time to come. It brought tears to her eyes. (Note: a copy of that letter was placed in the nurse's permanent file.)

The director's action so impressed me that I telephoned her the following day. I thought she should know the impact her action had on that workshop group. She was delighted to get positive feedback. Her letter-writing campaign was a new venture inspired by her motto: "Happy nurses mean happy patients."

Penny-pinching institutions should be reminded that the least expensive and most effective recruiting is done by satisfied employees. Happy employees enthusiastically recommend their employer to friends and neighbors, colleagues and classmates. Other successful "recruiters" are satisfied patients, board members, and auxiliary volunteers who sing praises to the professionals they meet.

The most expensive and least effective way to recruit is through classified advertisements whether they are placed in newspapers, professional journals, or trade magazines. Even using commercial head-hunting agencies is more productive and less expensive.

Of course, some ads are more imaginative and more effective than others. Denver General Hospital reduced their RN vacancies from 50 to 6 with a campaign built around the theme "put yourself on the edge of excellence." Instead of the hit-and-miss recruitment programs many hospitals conduct, Denver General analyzed its product, defined target consumers, appraised their competition, and hit the bull's-eye.

Ads aimed at herds rarely produce the desired results. Any recruiter worth her salt knows ad campaigns must be directed toward specific targets. A worthy recruiter also knows the best targets.

Nursing students about to enter the labor market for the first time are ready recruits. They should be vigorously courted and eased into their first professional assignment gently. If your facility develops a reputation as a good place to launch a career, you can have the cream of the crop from any nursing school.

If you abuse new graduates, giving them too much too soon, you will develop a reputation as a bad place to launch a career. The cream of the crop will go elsewhere. You'll get the leftovers.

Another prime target are people who call or write the hospital for information. They should be given first-class attention. What about nurses who walk in unannounced? Roll out the red carpet! They have made the first move, the next move is yours. First impressions can entice the potential staff member to take a closer look or send them running toward the nearest exit.

Now that the shortage has abated, will hospitals disband their recruitment and retention efforts? The smart ones won't. They will redouble their efforts because they know that their survival is linked both to the quantity and quality of nurses they hire.

Hospitals no longer have a blank check to cover their expenses and ensure their future. Cost containment is imperative. Institutions that are not fiscally fit will die. The mortality is expected to top 30 percent. That means more than 2000 hospitals will close. Will yours be one?

As has already been discussed, the cost of replacing nurses is prohibitive. Dollars invested in successful retention programs will pay for themselves a hundredfold.

Just as hospitals cannot afford to replace nurses, they cannot afford to hire the wrong nurses. Herds of nurses just passing through (floats, rentals, and novices) can spell financial disaster. Today, more than ever, things have to be done right the first time. With the advent of DRGs, a high-quality staff will pay for itself. A low-quality staff will put the hospital out of business.

As hospitals scramble for survival, the demand for herds will be down and heads up!

CHAPTER 5
Prolonging Professional Life

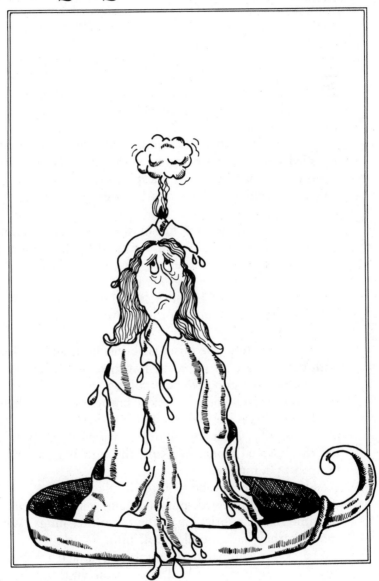

For years Sally had worked at a large state institution. The staffing was poor, the equipment archaic, the leadership lethargic, and the patients chronic.

For several months she had been feeling increasingly irritable and fatigued. Her optimism had been slowly replaced by a nagging pessimism. She had begun to question the institution's priorities, psychiatry's usefulness, the patients' progress, nursing's future, and her own competence.

Only two things kept her on the job: a fading sense of duty and overwhelming inertia. When she tried to discuss her feelings with colleagues, they were either too busy or too frustrated themselves to listen.

A classic case of burnout, wouldn't you say? You and I both know all the signs and symptoms. Burnout is easy to spot—in other people.

Unfortunately, the onset is so insidious and gradual, the person with the "disease" is often the last to know. That's why it is so important to have good friends, colleagues, and supervisors who can sense trouble and send help before burnout extinguishes your career.

In Sally's case burnout was cured in a dramatic and highly unorthodox way. Near midnight, after a particularly trying shift, she left the hospital alone. Walking through the parking lot, she was jumped by a mugger.

She beat the bejeebers out of him!

She kicked, clawed, punched, and generally walloped him. All the time she was shrieking at the top of her lungs. When help came running, they had to pull *her* off him.

Later she compared the mugger's attack to shock therapy. It jolted her out of apathy and into action. In those few moments, all her pent-up anger and frustration were released.

Suddenly energized, she began to evaluate her professional future. She realized she wasn't doing anyone a favor by staying in her present position.

Three weeks later she took a new job in a community mental health center. Her energy, optimism, and creativity returned. Once again she began enjoying work instead of enduring it.

"Enduring" work is one warning signal of impending burnout. Other signs and symptoms might include:

Irritability	No sense of purpose	Smoking more
Impatience		Drinking more
	Bitching	
Fatigue		Eating more
	Boredom	
Exhaustion		Feeling guilty
	Malaise	
Depression		Dreading work
	Whining	
Cynicism		Apathy
	Weeping	
Pessimism		Loneliness
	Poor concentration	
Loss of idealism		Uncooperativeness
	Indecisiveness	
Carelessness		Paralyzed creativity
	Feeling helpless	
Playing hookey		Denial
	Feeling powerless	
Being tardy		Rationalization
	Callousness	
Aches and pains		Insomnia

Usually before you burn out, you have to burn up. Anger, frustration, and righteous indignation are not uncommon predecessors. Your professional survival depends on what you do with that anger. Anger is energy. Channeled properly, changes can be made and burnout averted.

If you absorb the anger instead of harnessing it, the result is depression. There is no energy in depression. There is only resignation: "What's the use? Who cares? I give up."

Who are the people most susceptible to burnout? The best and the brightest. Hardworking idealists. Perfectionists.

Which jobs lend themselves most to burnout? Jobs in which constant high performance is required. Jobs in which expectations are unclear or unrealistic. Jobs in which workers have little control over what they do or how they do it. Demanding, stressful, people-related jobs. Jobs that couple overwhelming responsibility with powerlessness. Jobs that offer little financial reward, recognition, or appreciation.

Nursing fits the description. Nurses are prime candidates for burnout.

Although information about burnout is important, knowledge alone will not prevent it any more than knowledge will prevent disease. Knowledge is a tool. Unless you pick up the tool and use it to change your professional life-style, it is worthless.

If you want to save your professional life, here are a half-dozen suggestions:

Learn to Pace Yourself

Many burnout victims approach their career as though it were a 100-yard dash instead of a multimile marathon. Quickly caught up in the frenzy around them, they dash from crisis to crisis.

Perhaps they really believe that by working harder and longer, they can get everyone well. Then, and only then, will they sit down and take a break.

Professionals like that never get a break. They just get broken.

Take Care of Yourself

If you don't take care of yourself, no one else will. Eat right. Get enough rest. Exercise regularly. Be kind to yourself.

Fence off a few minutes each day just to reflect and dream in solitude. Forget the boss, patients, spouse, children, in-laws. Take time to renew yourself physically, mentally, emotionally, and spiritually. Private time is not a luxury. It's a necessity.

Learn to Leave Work Behind

Don't let work preempt your personal life. Socialize. Protect your family time.

Be aware of how work can contaminate your personal life. Alice is a good example of this problem. She had worked almost 3 years in neonatal intensive care. Originally she and her husband, Steve, had planned to save for a house and then have children. They both loved children.

Financially secure and house in hand, Steve was surprised when Alice suddenly refused to have children. Actually, it wasn't a sudden decision at all. It wasn't even a conscious decision. The daily dose of pain, death, and disability of her tiny patients and their distraught parents had subtly taken its toll. Alice was no longer anxious to have children. She was terrified.

The marriage nearly collapsed before Alice got the help she needed. Fortunately, the hospital had an excellent psychiatrist available to the staff and an active peer counseling program. A change of assignment and some intense, individual therapy helped Alice regain a healthy perspective.

Today, with two thriving children of her own, Alice is thinking of returning to neonatal ICU. She feels her maturity and positive personal experiences have made her strong enough to again tackle that difficult assignment.

Some experts think non-work-related activities are the key to preventing burnout. That poses a special problem for women whose professional duties are often an extension and refinement of what they do at home: cook, clean, comfort, etc.

To effectively separate your personal and professional life, you may need some decompression time between work and home. Jog, dance, garden, swim, or sauna. Participate in activities that clear your mind and refresh your spirit. Don't be surprised if you have to *work* at relaxation.

Activate Assertiveness Skills

Take the initiative. Make choices not excuses. Ask for what you need. Ask for what you want.

Say "no" to double shifts, 7-day stretches, and duties sloughed by impertinent physicians and uncooperative colleagues.

Say "yes" to the nursing activities you thoroughly enjoy. Make good use of the 80/20 principle by remembering that 80 percent of the pleasure you derive from nursing will come from completing 20 percent of your duties.

Identify the duties that give you the most satisfaction. One way to do this is to complete the following sentence in as many ways as possible:

"I feel very satisfied when I leave work knowing _____

_____

_____

_____."

49

Here are some examples from other nurses:

"I feel very satisfied when I leave work knowing:
I handled interpersonal problems tactfully."
the families' needs have been met."
the charts are complete."
the utility rooms are clean."
the medications were given on time."
I listened carefully."
the patients are better informed."
I learned something new."
I used my knowledge and skill to the best of my ability."
I was super efficient."
the next shift has the information and supplies needed."
I have made *one* patient more comfortable."

You will never *find* time to do the things you enjoy most in nursing. You have to *make* time for them. Maximize your professional satisfaction by indulging in your favorite nursing activities daily. Satisfied nurses don't burn out.

Optimize Time Management

Simplify. Set priorities. Delegate.

Clarify your values. Set goals and direct your activities toward their achievement.

Spend time wisely. Invest it. Don't squander it on people or activities unless they are really important to you.

Respect Your Humanness

You're only human. That's your greatest strength and your greatest weakness.

Resist unrealistic demands from within or without. Don't succumb! Don't be a dodo (Dead On Duty Overdose).

Burnout is contagious. Look closely at your professional companions. When you leave their company, do you feel refreshed and energized or drained and disillusioned?

Andrea, a struggling student nurse, seemed slated for failure. Suddenly she showed great improvement in her academic work. Her clinical performance also improved dramatically.

When her instructor complimented her and asked what had made such a difference, Andrea replied, "Oh, I just switched tables."

Week after week she had sat at the same table in the cafeteria surrounded by students who were also floundering academically and clinically. They spent the lunch hour moaning and complaining.

One noon, during a lengthy tirade by a disgruntled companion, Andrea's attention wandered. She noticed another table where the students were smiling, laughing, and talking excitedly about their experiences. The next day Andrea switched tables.

By the end of the week she began to feel more confident and capable. Soon she no longer questioned her ability to make it in nursing. She was sure she could!

Sometimes you have to fight to save your professional life. Sometimes you have to switch. You may need to switch tables, shifts, units, assignments, hospitals, or jobs. Ideally you won't have to switch careers.

◆　◆　◆

When colleagues begin to flicker and dim, what can you do to help? Encourage them to take a break, minivacation, or mental health day. Listen without being judgmental. Help them identify choices, options, and alternatives. Support their decisions.

Be empathetic. Smile. Say "please" and "thank you." Talk to them. Encourage *esprit de corps.* Invite them to join you at a stress-reduction workshop.

Help them increase their skills in problem solving, time management, and assertiveness. Give positive feedback. Encourage a change in assignment, responsibilities, shifts, or units. Stand up for them. Be there.

Preventive maintenance is as important for people as it is for machinery. Both can burn out if used excessively or improperly.

If you are a manager, whether first-time team leader or well-worn director of nursing, you can help save the professional lives of the people who work for you. Here are some tips:

- Assign where they can shine . . . where they can succeed.
- Make policies and procedures clear.
- Clarify role expectations.
- Define realistic goals for work output.
- Strengthen problem-solving and time-management skills.

51

- Provide an atmosphere of sharing and cohesiveness.
- Be flexible.
- Listen.
- Encourage.
- Praise.
- Provide individual counseling or a support group.
- Encourage growth and development.
- Individualize orientation.
- Don't expect perfection.
- Allow the individual as much control over her own work as possible.
- Encourage wellness activities.
- Maintain consistency.
- Allow direct, honest communication—without reprisals.
- Infuse with energy and enthusiasm.

If you want to know how to keep your nurse-employees on the job, don't ask the experts, ask your nurses themselves. When I suggest this to managers, they panic. They are sure nurses will immediately ask for more money.

Lack of communication between employers and employees often leads to misinformation and mismanagement. In one study the top six working conditions employees said they wanted were:

1. Interesting work
2. Full appreciation of work done
3. Feeling of being in on things
4. Job security
5. Good pay
6. Promotion and growth

At the same time the top six working conditions their employers *thought* the employees wanted were:

1. Good pay
2. Job security
3. Promotion and growth
4. Good working conditions
5. Interesting work
6. Tactful discipline

If you're still afraid the people who work for you are totally mercenary, try asking them what they want other than higher salaries. I have been asking nurses this question:

> What could your employer do for you, other than offering you more money, to increase your loyalty to the institution and ensure your continued employment?

Although there is some overlapping, most responses fall into six categories: (1) respect, (2) autonomy and opportunity, (3) communication, (4) management style and decision making, (5) education, and (6) financial considerations (suggestions that would cost money). Let me share some quotes with you:

Respect
"Be loyal to me."
"Support me with administration, physicians, and staff."
"Give us the same respect and consideration given doctors."
"Care about my feelings and ideas."
"Treat me fairly."
"Recognize my skills."
"Respect my education and experience."
"Treat me like a professional."
"Let me interview employees for my unit *before* their hiring."
"Provide reserved parking space."
"Stand behind me."
"Trust me."
"Give the nursing staff more say."
"Give praise for a job well done."

Autonomy and Opportunity
"Allow me to work freely with ideas."
"Let me follow through on projects I start."
"When you give me a job, let *me* find the best way to do it."
"Make me feel like I'm trusted. Don't stand over me all the time."
"Unless I've shown that I'm incompetent, decrease *control* over my activities."
"Give me authority over my own work."
"Provide more support for individual advancement."
"Help me grow in managerial skills."
"Let me know I can advance."
"Allow me freedom to make changes."

"Provide room for intellectual and emotional growth."
"Let me be free to create."
"Promote me!!!"

Communication

"Face-to-face, one-on-one meetings with my supervisor each
  week."
"Listen to my suggestions."
"Keep me informed *before* something changes."
"Encourage us—cheer us on!"
"Give positive feedback . . . occasionally . . . please?"
"Say 'thanks.' "
"Listen. Act when necessary."
"Increase direct, honest communication."
"Talk to *me!*"
"Be truthful."
"Consult us 'little guys' before changing policies."
"Provide more contact with other shifts."

Management style and decision making

"Be fair."
"Lead and guide instead of push."
"Give me bite-sized pieces to work on."
"Be receptive and friendly."
"Support my interests and projects."
"Involve us in management."
"Support my decisions."
"Help problem solve."
"Follow through!"
"Give fair, productive evaluations."
"Less confusion and more organization so I know what my job is."
"Be open to suggestion."
"Consistent personnel policies."
"Not on call 24 hours a day, 7 days a week."
"Provide adequate staffing. Not just in numbers but in quality as
  well."
"When it comes to the department I run, let me be the real decision
  maker."
"Have the people who work directly in patient care involved in
  decisions."
"Let us choose the supplies and equipment that we use daily."
"Give me freedom to make decisions appropriate for my position."

Education

"Grant time off for continuing education."

"Provide BSN and MSN classes in hospital."

"Increase educational opportunities."

"Reward academic achievement."

"Allow a schedule flexible enough, so I can pursue a degree."

"Unless the hospital is willing to put up the money and free up my time, they should get off my back about getting a degree."

Financial considerations

"Raise my salary."

"Increase benefits."

"Fully paid health, dental, and life insurance."

"In-house child care."

"Make three 12-hour shifts full time."

"No layoffs."

"More overtime."

"Better retirement."

"$100 deductible rather than $300."

"Free tuition."

"Enough equipment to do the job."

"Give us a lounge and cafeteria equal to the one provided for doctors."

There were also numerous requests for better hours, more weekends and holidays off, and flexible schedules. As one nurse put it, "I'd give anything to get a schedule more congruent with my life."

◆ ◆ ◆

In conclusion, pause and take a good look at yourself. Professionally speaking, are you alive or just lingering? Are the people who work with you or for you thriving or barely surviving?

If the quality of your professional life is questionable, prolonging it may be a grave disservice. There are worse things than death for a person or a professional. If you have to make a choice, go for quality.

CHAPTER 6

Profit and Loss

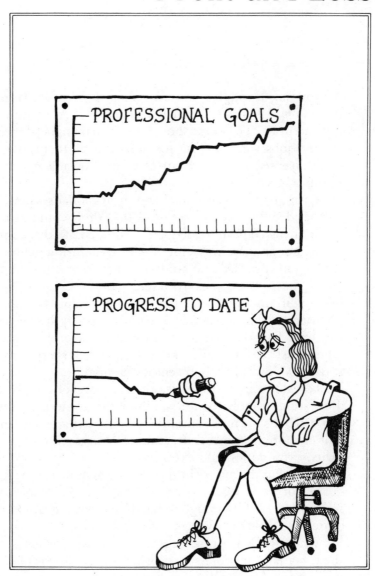

$\mathbf{B}$rowsing through a souvenir shop, I spotted a large button that read, *"I'm depressed—no one is after my job."* At the time it was painfully accurate. The nurse shortage was making headlines. While over 100,000 jobs were waiting for nurses to fill them, over 300,000 actively licensed registered nurses were choosing not to work in the health care system.

For a myriad of personal and professional reasons, those nurses had decided they would lose more than they would gain by working. Their *profits* could not adequately compensate them for their *losses*.

Although there was a lot of talk about luring old nurses back and enticing new students to study nursing, it was just that—talk. And talk is cheap. Even in excruciating shortages, nurses' salaries, working conditions, and fringe benefits don't improve dramatically.

Many claim nurses are not motivated by monetary incentives. Just once I would like to see hospitals make offers nurses couldn't refuse. Just once I would like to see night nurse positions advertised at $40,000 instead of a 40 cent differential.

For some mysterious reason the laws of supply and demand don't seem to apply to nurses. I think the mysterious reason is *Rubber Nurse*. That's the nurse employers can stretch to cover more than one unit or more than one shift. Rubber Nurses (RNs) take on extra patients, extra duties, and extra days.

Believing the nurse shortage is real and not just a figment of low salaries or poor working conditions, Rubber Nurses work longer and harder. Pliable enough to handle everything from orthopedics to obstetrics, RNs can even pass for ICU nurses in a pinch.

When Rubber Nurse begins to lose her elasticity, she is chided about her lack of professional commitment. She is blackmailed with suggestions that her lack of flexibility endangers patients' welfare. Ironically it is her fatigue and her acceptance of assignments exceeding her competence that really endanger patients.

Eventually the paycheck, the pat on the back, the impassioned calls to duty are no longer enough to keep Rubber Nurse bouncing back for more. Stretched beyond her limits, she finally snaps. She bounces right out of her job and/or her profession. The cost of staying has become prohibitive. Her losses exceed her profits.

You and I have invested heavily in nursing. We have put a lot of time, money, and energy into our profession. As young nurses, few of us ever thought about what financial return there would be on such investments.

A 20-year veteran of the nursing profession vividly recalls receiving her first paycheck. When she opened her envelope, she was very disappointed at the amount enclosed. As a student, it never occurred to her to ask about potential salary. When she applied for her first job, she was so excited about being hired, she had not even thought to ask.

Even today women often neglect to ask important financial questions when considering jobs or careers. Laura was one would-be nurse who asked questions and got unexpected answers.

Having been disappointed in her marriage, Laura decided to make one of her other dreams come true. Since childhood, she wanted to become a nurse. Armed with resolve, she went to her nearby community college and made the necessary inquiries.

Unfortunately, her science and math background was so meager it would take a full year just to meet prerequisites for entrance. There were already so many qualified applicants the college had resorted to a lottery to choose students. *If* she were lucky enough to be selected on her first try, she could complete all her studies in 3 years.

Although it would be difficult to support herself and two children during those years, Laura thought she could manage. She was willing to put forth any effort and make many sacrifices. That is, she was willing until she had a frank talk with a nursing faculty advisor. At that point Laura had a rather rude awakening. She had never thought about the realities of *being* a nurse. She had only dreamed of *becoming* a nurse.

For the past 5 years Laura had worked as a toll collector on an interstate bridge. One aspect of her job that she found most distressing was having to rotate shifts and work some holidays and weekends. When the faculty advisor spelled out local hospital policies, Laura was surprised to discover her working conditions were superior to those of nurses. In fact, given her present salary, working conditions, fringe benefits, and future prospects, it was immediately clear that Laura could not afford to be a nurse.

Yes, she was disappointed. All dreams die hard. Little-girl dreams of marriage. Little-girl dreams of careers.

Can *you* afford to be a nurse?

Even the most charitable societies and institutions have begun to admit their survival depends on their ability to turn a profit. They realize profits must not only cover today's expenses but tomorrow's as well. For without sufficient profits there will be no tomorrow.

Profit is not a necessary evil. Profit is simply necessary. When a service or product ceases to be profitable, it ceases to exist.

To survive, any business must be able to cover costs. To *thrive,* a business must do much more. Thriving means having funds for expansion; for education, research, and development; for repairing, replacing, and upgrading equipment; and for meeting rising costs of personnel, goods, and services.

It is almost sacrilegious to link profit and nursing. The thought that we "profit" from others' illnesses and misfortunes seems almost obscene. Yet that is exactly what we do. We fill a vital need, and in return we are paid for our services. *Caring* is our business.

Can nursing accept its need to be profitable? Can you?

Nurses have always been a bit like dethroned royalty—poor but proud. We find discussions of money crude. We prefer to focus on tradition, service, sacrifice, duty, and honor. Those are noble words. But if nursing is to survive and thrive, we must also focus on words like recognition, respect, success, and solvency.

As one nurse so succinctly put it, "Nursing is a great life but a crummy living."

Making nursing both a good life *and* a good living will not be easy.

A couple of years ago, I interviewed a woman welder. After 10 years on the job, she was making $20 an hour. Even an apprentice welder, just out of high school and not knowing which end of the blow torch to use, made $10 an hour. At that very same time nurses' salaries ranged from $6 to $7.50 an hour.

The first blow is to realize nurses are worth less than welders. The second blow is to realize that experience is more highly valued in welders than in nurses. An experienced welder is worth twice that of an inexperienced one. The same is not true for nurses.

Compressed salary scales continue to provide little reward for experienced nurses. In the May 1983 issue of *RN* magazine, an obviously startled nurse reported that when her hospital recently hired a new graduate, they discovered their new employee was making a mere $1000 less than her mother who's been a nurse with the hospital for over 15 years!

Commenting on this very common situation, professional nurse recruiter Chris Corbin wrote, "In most health care institutions, the registered nurse reaches the top of her salary scale in 5 to 7 years and thereafter receives only cost of living adjustments, if that."*

Actually, loyalty to a health care institution is rarely rewarded and often penalized. Taught that discussing salaries is "unprofessional," many experienced nurses have been slow to discover their salaries are less than those of newly employed, inexperienced nurses.

At the height of the nurse shortage, the Colorado legislature agreed to raise entry-level salaries to attract much-needed new nurses. Novices were soon being hired at salaries exceeding those of loyal, long-term nurse employees, not to mention those of their head nurses. The legislators seemed genuinely surprised by the uproar that followed.

Many hospitals shy away from publishing definite salary figures when advertising for nurses. They resort to euphemisms like "salary commensurate with experience and education." That empty phrase promises much more than it delivers.

How much is education worth? In their initial report the National Commission on Nursing says only about 12 percent of hospitals pay registered nurses with baccalaureate degrees more than those with lesser education.

Perhaps you work for one of the few institutions that does reward educational efforts. Knowing your hospital pays more for nurses with degrees may be one of the reasons you are thinking of going back to college. You may even be among the thousands of nurses already working toward degrees. Did you ever stop to ask your hospital exactly how much your degree will be worth?

Looking at the guides to career opportunities published annually by nursing journals is quite an eye-opener. Hospitals throughout the United States spend big money on full-page advertisements hoping to entice nurses like you to come and work for them. In the 1980 guides they offered everything from free laundry service to Hawaiian vacations.

---

*Solutions, RN **46**:34j, 1983.

As I reviewed their ads, I noticed some boasting a $300 differential for registered nurses with baccalaureate degrees. I was impressed. After all, $3600 per year is nothing to sneeze at. Then I noticed a $600 differential for nurses with master's degrees. I was doubly impressed.

All at once I realized they were not talking about a monthly differential. They were talking about a *yearly* differential. I was no longer impressed. I was depressed.

Picking $20,000 as a moderate cost for acquiring a baccalaureate degree, I did some quick calculations. If the hospitals were generous and gave you a dollar a day, it would take you 55 years to recoup your investment. Even picking $10,000 as the cost of that additional education, it would take you more than 27 years just to break even.

In *The AJN Guide: A Review of Nursing Career Opportunities in 1982,*★ Michael Reese Hospital in Chicago advertises that ADN-diploma graduates are paid $8.98 per hour whereas BSN graduates receive $9.15 per hour. If you work for them, your baccalaureate degree will be worth 17 cents per hour. Seventeen cents!

How much is experience worth? Let's get down to brass tacks. In that same guide Cedars-Sinai Medical Center in Los Angeles advertises, "New graduates start between $19,136 and $20,093, while experienced RNs can expect to start between $20,093 and $21,091." Your experience is worth roughly $1000 or 5 percent. Obviously nurses don't get better, just older.

Of course, there are reasons other than financial gain to pursue higher education. Education often unlocks doors to job opportunities providing more personal and professional satisfaction.

Actually, the satisfactions of the nursing profession are seldom measured in terms of dollars or "sense." Nurses defy logic by continuing to work in spite of physical strain, emotional drain, and lack of tangible rewards.

An advertising executive has a plaque on her wall that reads:

"In the ad game,
the days are tough,
the nights are long,
and the work is emotionally demanding.

★O'Connor, Andrea B., editor: The AJN guide: a review of nursing career opportunities in 1982, New York, 1982, American Journal of Nursing Company.

But it's all worth it,
because the rewards
   are shallow,
    transparent,
and meaningless."

In the nursing game the days are tough, the nights are long, and the work is emotionally demanding. But it's all worth it *because* of the rewards. The rewards may be intangible, but they are far from being shallow, transparent, or meaningless.

If you have ever gotten misty eyed reading first-person accounts in professional journals about "my most unforgettable patient," you know what I am talking about. We've all had unforgettable patients. And one special patient, vividly remembered, can carry a nurse through the frustrations of long hours, poor staffing, and bizarre scheduling.

Nursing is rich in intangible rewards. Have you ever thought about which intangibles are most important to you?

During an after-dinner conversation at an interdisciplinary conference, a doctor and a nurse discovered they had both been offered top positions at a major metropolitan hospital. Since the hospital was about to launch a highly specialized intensive care department, it was in search of the best medical and nursing professionals it could find.

As the two discussed their interviews, experiences, and observations, I listened intently. Both were struck by the magnitude of the project and intrigued by the challenge it promised. Both found the city appealing. Both mentioned the young, inexperienced staff that was in great need of guidance from seasoned professionals.

It was the hospital's great need that most impressed the nurse. She was obviously struggling with her decision to accept or reject the hospital's offer.

Although the doctor also acknowledged the hospital's great need, he did not feel compelled to donate himself to their cause. He had already made his reply to the hospital's offer. He had declined.

Encouraging her to consider her own needs, not just the hospital's, the doctor said, "I know they will be extremely fortunate to get you. I just wonder if you will be equally fortunate to get them. Have you thought about what *you* will gain from this experience?"

The doctor went on to share his primary reason for declining the position. The hospital could not offer him what he valued most: first-rate peers. He had discovered the synergistic effect of working shoulder-to-shoulder with top-notch professionals. If he took the new position, he could give a lot to the young staff, but the kinds of things they could give him in return would not enhance his productivity. In his present position he enjoyed developing young staff, but he also enjoyed being surrounded by accomplished professionals who matched or exceeded his talent, intellect, curiosity, and drive.

How easy it is to forget our own needs when others' needs clamor for our attention! How difficult it is to maintain the proper balance between nourishing others and being nourished ourselves!

Striving to match our qualifications to the needs of the institution, we are often distracted from asking an equally important question: *do the institution's qualifications match our needs?*

Just how well are *your* needs being met by the institution for which you work? Considering everything from your present performance to your future prospects, how satisfied are you with your current job? Ask yourself the following questions:

1. Do I look forward to going to work each day?
2. Do I leave work feeling satisfied and successful?
3. What new skill or insight have I acquired this past week? Month? Year?
4. What old skill or knowledge have I mastered?
5. What one thing did I accomplish this week that will have lasting value?
6. What outstanding piece of nursing did I do this past week? Month? Year?
7. How am I using this job to meet my short-term goals? Long-term goals?
8. How will this job make me a better nurse?
9. Which of my fringe benefits do I consider most valuable?
10. Does my salary reflect my experience, education, and level of responsibility?
11. What are my opportunities for advancement in the next 12 months?
12. How would I describe the people I work with shoulder-to-shoulder each day? (Choose up to four words from the following list to describe them.)

WORD LIST	PEOPLE WORKING WITH ME

WORD LIST

Informed
Supportive
Innovative
Fair
Creative
Decisive
Spirited
Intelligent
Caring
Professional
Trustworthy
Honest
Reliable
Organized
Hard working
Humanitarian
Efficient
Effective
Generous
Skillful
Ambitious
Enthusiastic

PEOPLE WORKING WITH ME

Nurses
1. _____
2. _____
3. _____
4. _____

Doctors
1. _____
2. _____
3. _____
4. _____

Supervisors
1. _____
2. _____
3. _____
4. _____

Administrators
1. _____
2. _____
3. _____
4. _____

Other personnel
1. _____
2. _____
3. _____
4. _____

To survive in any job you need adequate amounts of:

FINANCIAL REWARD
INTELLECTUAL STIMULATION
EMOTIONAL SATISFACTION

To thrive, you need optimal amounts.

If you do not find your job financially rewarding, intellectually stimulating, and/or emotionally satisfying, it is time to find a new job. If you do not find the nursing profession financially rewarding, intellectually stimulating, and/or emotionally satisfying, it is time to find a new profession. *Or* it is time to do something to make your job and profession more "profitable" in the tangible and intangible ways you value most.

There's a word I like to borrow from economics. Satisfice. It's a combination of two words: satisfy and sacrifice. Satisfice is that point at which the satisfaction achieved justifies the sacrifices involved.

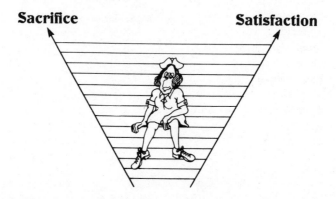

Sacrifice   **Satisfaction**

As you go onward and upward, you reach a level where you can live comfortably with the sacrifices and satisfactions life has to offer.

Great satisfaction usually involves great sacrifice. Ask any Olympic athlete or concert violinist. They sacrifice everything from careers to companionship in the single-minded pursuit of excellence.

Unfortunately, great sacrifice does not always ensure great satisfaction. You will find yourself in many ventures, jobs, and relationships that demand more from you than they are willing to give in return. A yard of sacrifice may only produce an inch of reward. You find yourself a victim of diminishing returns.

Sacrifice   **Satisfaction**

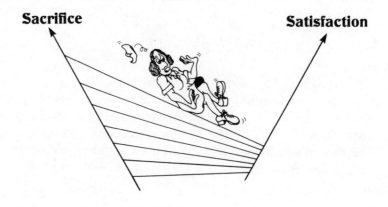

If the sacrifices greatly exceed the satisfactions, things can go downhill pretty fast.

Imagine for a moment that you have decided to be an Olympic-quality runner. Running becomes your life. It squeezes everything else out. It devours your time, energy, and money. You hire a coach, train constantly, buy special gear, and travel to competitions.

As a novice you don't expect to win right away, but you don't expect to lose consistently either. If you continue to trail behind, you may redouble your efforts. However, if your record still doesn't improve, you will probably be reluctant to invest any more time, energy, or money in the sport.

Eventually, discouraged by your lack of significant progress, you decide to cut your losses and run. Or rather, stop running. You either give it up altogether, or you become a recreational runner.

Years ago many of us dreamed of being Olympic-quality nurses. We trained hard and worked hard. We invested our time, energy, and money. Nursing became the center of our lives.

As novices we didn't expect big financial rewards or undue respect. We were willing to get additional coaching, training, and practice. Yet even after losing our amateur status, our profession still was not forthcoming with adequate rewards or recognition.

Thinking it was a personal problem and not a professional one, we redoubled our efforts. We got more education, took on new assignments, added responsibilities, switched into administration and education. Still the sacrifices demanded of us by our employers far exceeded our rewards.

Eventually, many of us decided to cut our losses and run. Nursing ceased to be the central focus of our lives. Some of us gave it up altogether. Others decided to become *Recreational Nurses*.

Recreational Nurses dabble in nursing. They no longer take their professional life too seriously. They like to keep a hand in nursing, but they have pulled their heads and hearts out. They work a day or two a week or donate time on the bloodmobile. Nursing provides a nice break from the other activities of their lives.

Rubber Nurses. Recreational Nurses. We are all RNs.

Sacrifice and satisfaction have tangible and intangible components. The tangible ones are more easily identified and calibrated. The intangible ones are highly individual.

Even though the tangible rewards nursing offers remain compressed, the opportunity for intangible rewards is greater than in most jobs or professions. Those intangibles—sense of purpose, involvement, humanitarian goals—lift the satisfaction level enough to justify the sacrifices we must make to remain active in nursing.

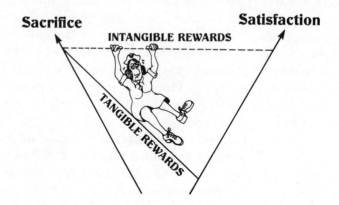

Clinging to those intangibles can help save your professional life.

Saving your professional life may require shoring up both your tangible and intangible rewards. For example, if you are not satisfied with your salary, ask for a raise. It is surprising how few nurses ever do.

A sudden gust of courage propelled one nurse into her supervisor's office. She blurted out her request for a raise. The good news is she got it. The bad news is that it only amounted to 15 cents an hour.

If you want to be more successful than she was, first do your homework. Here are some tips that may help you:

Inventory your skills, knowledge, and abilities.
Estimate your contribution to the organization's goals.
Know whether you are seen as disposable or indispensable.
Know the precedents.
Envision all possible reactions to your request.
Anticipate questions that might be asked. Rehearse answers.
Make a formal appointment.
Have a specific dollar figure in mind.
Smile. Radiate confidence.
Focus on your worth, not on your need.

If your salary is tied to all other nurses' salaries, individual raises may be out. Collective bargaining takes over.

Regarding collective bargaining, all I can say is nurses need **help!** Nothing in our backgrounds has prepared us to negotiate intelligently and boldly. Hire experts. Heed their advice.

A midwest director of nursing shared her disappointment with the outcome of recent negotiations at her hospital. As part of the management team, her attention and allegiance had to go to the greater goals of the organization. Yet she could not help feeling sad and frustrated as she watched the staff nurses settle for far less than the hospital was willing to offer.

Settling for less. Surviving but not thriving.

What will it take to satisfy you? Do you crave challenge, involvement, advancement, autonomy, support, first-class peers, flexible scheduling, new surroundings, better benefits, brighter prospects?

Everything is negotiable. You just have to decide what you want and what you are willing to sacrifice to get it. Ideally you won't have to sacrifice your profession.

CHAPTER 7

Prophet Sharing

Our satellite shows scattered hospices, frequent home births, and a possible increase in rehabilitation centers. Hospital per diem costs will reach highs of $400 and lows of $200. Gusts of old geezers are reported moving toward the southwest at speeds up to 55 mph. Film at eleven.

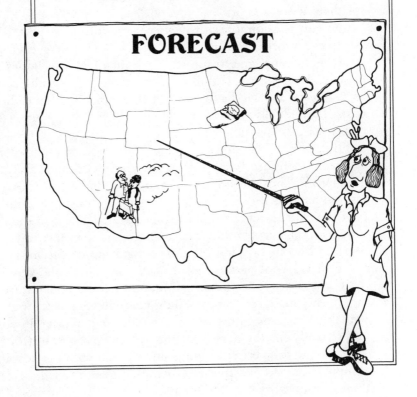

Attention ★ *K-Mart* ★ *Shoppers!* Under the flashing blue light in the center aisle you will find our nurse. For the next 5 minutes only, blood pressure readings half price."

A fantasy of the future? Not really. Health care clinics have already been established in many shopping malls. Some even provide patients with beepers to carry while they're shopping. Then, when the doctor is ready to see them, their beeper sounds, and they return for their appointment.

As competition for patients increases, you can expect to see more creative ventures. Hospitals are already offering everything from steak and champagne to money-back guarantees in hopes of luring patients. Everyone is scrambling for the vanishing health care dollar.

Collectively, we have all been screaming for lower health care costs. Individually, however, we still believe that when it comes to our *own* care, "Money is no object!"

But money is an object. You don't have to be much of a prophet to predict a future based on profit. Competition is already fierce. "For-profit" hospitals are siphoning off the well-endowed, well-insured patients leaving the "not-for-profit" hospitals with the indigent, uninsured patients. While one hospital grabs all the profitable obstetrical business, another corners the market on coronary care. A bonanza for one hospital may mean bankruptcy for another.

That may not be the way it *should* be. That's the way it *is*.

If you want to see nursing in the future and your future in nursing, open your eyes. The first thing you will see is a computer. When you think of computers, do you smile or grimace? If you smile, you're ready for the future. If you grimace, you're in trouble.

Two nurses were struggling side by side with the hospital's new computerized system. In total frustration one growled, "I've had it! I think I'll go work for 'St. Ignats.'" The other returned, "Haven't you heard? Their computer system will be on line in another 2 months."

In addition to being computerized, here's what some nurses predict nursing's future to be:

"Providing quantity of life without quality"
"Return to acute care"
"Teaching, planning, coordinating"
"*Intense* intensive care!"
"Independent, stressful, specialized"
"Management from afar—less actual patient involvement"
"Increasingly community oriented"
"More home health"
"More technical, less personal"
"Fanatic cost containment!"

Obviously nurses don't look too far into the future. Most of the items on this list were implemented yesterday.

Getting nurses to concentrate on the future isn't easy. We're too busy just getting through *today*. And, if tomorrow is anything like today, we'd rather not think about it at all.

Nurses tend to fight the future. We insist on swimming upstream. We complain, "The river shouldn't be running this way. It ought to run in the other direction."

Under great protest we are swept along. We cling to traditions, like rocks in a fast-moving stream, until the current overpowers us. We arrive in the future battered, bruised, exhausted . . . and late.

If we could learn to let go of the past and swim with the current, we might arrive in the future healthy, wealthy, wise . . . and on time.

Some of the things nurses say they would like to see in their future include:

"More control over the work situation"
"Better quality of life for patients"
"Promotion of wellness, independence, and self-care"
"Fewer 'housekeeping' tasks for nurses"
"Autonomy is a must!"
"Treating and educating patients as whole beings"
"Emphasis on prevention"
"Third-party payment"
"Salaries commensurate with expertise"
"Affordable, accessible health care"

When asked what they are doing to bring these things into being, they fall silent. Nurses need to learn that if they want to influence the future, they have to go where the future is being influenced.

For example, have you ever attended the board meeting at your hospital? Few nurses have. They are too busy giving bedbaths to bother with such stuff and nonsense. Unfortunately, while you're at the bedside, your future is being determined in the boardroom.

One way for nurses and nursing to stay viable is to figure out what consumers will want and need in the future. A good starting point is to examine the products and services available today. Which ones are lacking in quality or quantity?

What do health care consumers want? Exasperated nurses moan that patients want everything from "mind reading" to "maid service." Patients want "150 percent of my time and attention." Patients say, "Fix me—but I don't want to have to do anything to help myself." Another writes, "Champagne on a beer budget."

Some nurses see the burgeoning elderly population as a problem. Others see it as an opportunity. Workshop groups have lively discussions about future business opportunities for nursing in areas like elderly day care, intermediate care (between hospital and home or nursing home), in-the-home nursing, educational programs aimed at the elderly, preventive health packages including nutritional and social programs.

Nurses think health care consumers lack information both in quantity and quality. They see a need for:

"Adequate information on drugs and their use"
"Honest advertising"
"Interpreters of medical jargon"
"Truly informed consent"
"Better teaching concerning diagnosis, treatment alternatives, life-style adjustments"
"Adequate, accurate explanations of invasive procedures"
"Understandable information"
"More health maintenance information"
"Information on credibility of doctors—which are really the best?"
"Better hospital orientation, clearer information, more choice"
"Knowledge of medications in layman's terms"
"Diet *how*'s and *why*'s"

"Information on prices"
"Better understanding of where a health care dollar goes"
"Awareness of extent to which doctors regulate and control the
    system"
"Facts!"

Does this list suggest any future opportunities to you? If not,
try the next list. It centers on providing "quality" service. Nurses
feel health care consumers have a desire or need for:

"Better quality emergency room care"
"Privacy, self-respect, dignity"
"Personalized attention"
"Caring! Treatment as human beings"
"Discharge planning that provides enough support for wellness
    instead of just meeting the needs of illness"
"More time"
"Psychological support"
"Counseling"
"Access to modern techniques and knowledge"
"Respect for their time—less waiting!"
"Sense of continuity"
"Mutual respect between client and provider"
"Care planned to meet their needs, not the doctor's needs"
"Protection of patient's rights"
"Give choices"
"Listen!"
"Understanding . . . compassion . . . comfort . . . security"
"Top priority"
"Hospice"
"Involvement in decision making"
"Optimal care"
"The right to sexual activity in acute care setting"
"Attention!"

If nurses can provide "quality care with no frills and low bills,"
our future seems assured.

Jobs for nurses have usually been plentiful. One of the most attractive things about our profession has been the ability to find work
anytime, anywhere. After years of having more jobs than nurses, the
reverse is suddenly true. Jobs are scarce.

Feast or famine? In either event your professional future depends on your ability to find the best job possible. If it's a matter of survival, any job may be the right job. If you're more concerned with "thrival," you will have to be more creative and ingenious than ever before.

In the best of times or the worst of times, a job-hunting nurse needs a sound resume. That resume should include:

Name, address, and phone number
Educational experience
Work experience
Special skills or certifications
States in which licensed
Professional organizations

The resume should be concise, clear, clean, complete, and kept to a single page. Some nurses find it difficult to confine their resume to one page, whereas others complain theirs would fit on a postage stamp. If your career is lengthy and varied, select highlights and offer more details on request. If your resume is too thin, expand on job titles by including descriptions of activities or duties performed. You might also add personal interests or continuing education seminars attended to round out a full page.

When constructing your resume, maximize your assets. Don't overlook them. Take credit for your achievements. Use only positive words and phrases. Make use of action verbs like improved, implemented, directed, administered, supervised, taught, prepared, conducted, established, planned, and evaluated.

Do not list references on your resume. Offer them upon request after you are sure there is mutual interest between you and the prospective employer.

A cover letter should accompany your resume. Although the resume remains constant, the cover letter is personalized for each situation. It might include how you found out about the opening, why you are interested in the position, and the skills and qualities you possess that make you well suited to their needs. The tone should be confident and enthusiastic, so the recruiter or director will be enticed into granting an interview.

When preparing for the interview, find out everything possible about the position, the institution, and the person conducting the interview.

Ask yourself if you are just looking for work (survival) or trying to make a career-connected move (thrival).

Rehearse responses to possible questions like: Why do you want to change jobs? What were your duties in your last job? Why do you want this particular job? What is your nursing philosophy? And the ever popular, "Tell me about yourself."

Make a list of concrete examples demonstrating your ability to work efficiently and effectively. Concentrate on your strengths. Practice wording everything, including your shortcomings, in a positive manner.

Carry a notepad and pen with you. Bring along a list of questions you will want answered before making a decision. Take an extra copy of your resume and a list of three professional references including name, title, address, and phone number.

Dress in a conservative, professional manner. Don't smoke or chew gum.

Arrive on time or just moments before the scheduled appointment. Smile. Walk tall. Speak in a well-modulated voice. Maintain eye contact. Be friendly, respectful, and attentive. Exude confidence.

To decrease your nervousness during the interview try remembering this is a two-way street. Yes, they are interviewing you, but you are also interviewing them.

If at all possible visit the institution a few days before the interview and take a long, leisurely look around. Survey the grounds. Spend time eavesdropping in the cafeteria. Ask directions from different staff members. You can quickly assess whether this is an institution where people thrive or fight to survive.

Make your own observations. How confident, enthusiastic, and professional is the person conducting the interview? How well prepared is she? Is she evasive? Vague? Authoritarian? Would you like to work with or for this person?

Let the interviewer guide the session. Answer questions honestly and candidly. If a question takes you by surprise, don't feel compelled to blurt out an answer. Tell the interviewer you would like to give it some thought. Ask permission to come back to that question later.

When your turn comes to ask questions, consult your list. Inquire about patient care assignments, philosophies, staffing policies, continuing education opportunities, and advancement possibilities.

Finally, if the information hasn't already been offered, ask about salary, scheduling or shift requirements, and fringe benefits.

At the close of the interview, summarize your intent, interests, and hopes. If you are definitely not interested in the position, say so as tactfully as possible. If you are very interested, convey that message clearly. Negotiate a definite time frame in which they will let you know about the position or you will let them know about your decision.

If they offer you the job right on the spot, chances are they are desperate. If you accept right on the spot, you are desperate. Take your time, or you may be taken.

Follow up the interview with a brief thank-you note. Even if this position doesn't work out, there may be attractive future openings coming up. Your note will help them remember you as a very professional person with a lot of potential.

Are you prepared for future employment in nursing? Do you know where the jobs will most likely be? Predicted boom areas include hospice units and hospital-based in-home services. Other areas expected to grow rapidly include rehabilitation, oncology, IV therapy, orthopedics, and ambulatory units.

The larger the hospital, the more likely a BSN degree will be required in the near future. Nurses with special certification will also be in demand. Openings for "generic" nurses may decrease as demand for specialized nurses increases.

Is there a promotion in your future? That will probably depend on your willingness to obtain a degree and get special certification. Hard work is rarely the key to a promotion. The key is visibility—having the people at the top recognize you and your ability.

In first-rate institutions promotions go to those who are self-motivated, confident, eager, and ambitious. In second-rate institutions promotions go to those who are long-suffering, submissive, and compliant. First-rate institutions are more concerned with results. Second-rate ones focus on efforts. To determine which kind of institution you are in, look up the organizational ladder at least two or three rungs.

Good jobs are so hard to find, you may have to go out and create one. Today more than ever before, nurses are being forced to get their act together and take it on the road. Here is one nurse's success story:

One year ago on a dark and bleak Friday afternoon in April, my position, along with four of my colleagues', was suddenly dissolved. Wiped out of existence! Kaputt! We were all given until September to either find new positions in our institution or obtain positions elsewhere.

Well, after the shock and tears were over, determination set in. I decided I was good for my institution and I could make a place for myself. I was going to help my institution in spite of itself!

Gaining the support of one of my displaced colleagues, I began to tackle the problem. For a long time it had been my premise that our education department could support its in-house activities by marketing its resources to outside institutions.

First, I did the necessary field research. I visited outlying agencies and assessed their needs. I took a couple of business courses including one specifically geared to health care marketing. Then I wrote a marketing proposal (the first ever written at our "sophisticated" institution).

My colleague and I presented our proposal to the administrator. *It was approved and funded as a pilot project!!!*

Our pilot project lasted 6 months. I evaluated the data then revised the marketing objectives and plans. I presented the evaluation to the administrator myself. Again I passed inspection and the project was continued. Success!

If the project flops tomorrow, it doesn't matter. I have learned so much. It was scary at times and loads of work. But I made many new contacts, mastered moving things through red tape, and learned whom to work with and whom to work around.

This experience, which began as a horrible problem (complete with tears), ended as my greatest career opportunity. If my old job hadn't been "dissolved," I would have missed a lot of fun, excitement, and stimulation. I would never have become the knowledgeable, confident professional I am today.

Whether you like it or not, the future arrives daily. You can resist it, or you can run forward to meet it. The way the future is approached is what separates nurses who survive from those who thrive.

Welcome to the future!

CHAPTER 8

Procrastination

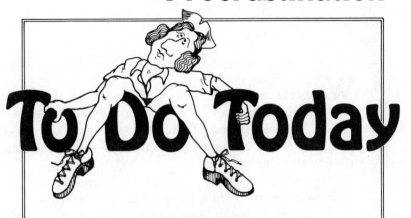

CRITICAL

1. _____   4. _____

2. _____   5. _____

3. _____   6. _____

Significant others   ## Insignificant others

_____   _____

_____   _____

_____   _____

_____   _____

_____   _____

_____   _____

_____   _____

_____   _____

While revising *STAT: Special Techniques in Assertiveness Training for Women in the Health Professions,* ★ I expanded the annotated bibliography. Reviewing one of the new additions titled "Overcoming Procrastination," I facetiously wrote, "I haven't gotten around to reading this one yet."

It was true. I owned the book for 3 years before I finally read it. Like many people I am an inveterate procrastinator.

For example, when I began writing this book, the nurse shortage was already excruciating and seemed to be escalating daily. As I dawdled along, the economy collapsed, and the nurse shortage all but disappeared. Some of my best rantings and ravings had to be re-evaluated and, alas, rewritten. Procrastination often demands a high price.

To procrastinate is to put off doing something until a future time, to postpone or delay needlessly. It's perfectly normal. Everyone does it. Nobody *wants* to do it, but everyone does it.

The three most common reasons for procrastination are:

1. Not wanting to begin.
2. Not knowing where to begin.
3. Not knowing where to begin, even if you wanted to begin, which you don't.

What have you been putting off or needlessly delaying? Getting a physical examination, making a dental appointment, starting a diet, knitting a sweater, looking for a job, disciplining an employee, obtaining a divorce, writing an article, attending college?

Some of the above tasks are unpleasant. Some are overwhelming. Some are both unpleasant and overwhelming.

You may have lots of good ideas and even more good intentions, but somehow time keeps slipping away and you never quite get started . . . or finished.

★St. Louis, 1983, The C.V. Mosby Co.

Self-help books will tell you to follow something like these "simple" steps:

1. Set priorities.
2. Focus on one problem at a time.
3. Give yourself a deadline and stick to it.
4. Don't sidestep difficult problems.
5. Remember, only God is perfect.

Seems simple enough, doesn't it? What those self-help books fail to tell you is that you may require years of psychotherapy to accomplish any one of the above.

Take the first directive: set priorities. When you set priorities, you are required to make decisions. Not only do you have to decide what you are going to do, you have to decide what you are *not* going to do.

Women often lack the self-confidence to be decisive. Fearful of making the "wrong" decision, we hesitate to make any decision. We overlook the fact that not to decide is to decide. It is decision by default. If you delay a decision long enough, it will be made for you. "This offer expires at midnight."

We tend to see choices as right or wrong, black or white, all or nothing. Although some choices may prove better than others, few involve such extremes. However, all decisions do involve an element of risk, and, unfortunately, women view risk as entirely negative. Women avoid risk. Women avoid making decisions.

The next time you are faced with an important choice, try viewing it as an *opportunity* instead of a problem. Most of us seize opportunities. All of us avoid problems.

Procrastinators typically spend more time and energy inventing excuses than it would take to invent solutions. Do any of these sound familiar?

"I'm just not in a creative mood."
"I'll start first thing tomorrow."
"Because of circumstances beyond my control. . . ."
"If I can't do it right, I won't do it at all."
"Not tonight. I have a headache."
"As soon as I solve my other problems, I'll get right on it."
"All work and no play. . . ."
"I work better under pressure."

Exploring the root causes of your procrastination may be a fascinating pastime, but it won't solve the problem. Insight doesn't solve problems, *action* does.

Five-Minute Antidote for Inertia

Time-management experts recognize the biggest hurdle to overcome is inertia. The old saying about the longest journey beginning with a single step is the basis for the 5-minute plan. Here is a practically painless way to take that first step.

Strike a bargain with yourself. Agree to give some miserable task 5 minutes of your time. That's right—just 5 minutes. You can stand almost anything for that length of time.

Set a timer and begin. When the timer rings, you may quit. That's fine. You have kept your bargain.

Instead of quitting immediately, you may decide to work just 5 minutes more. Reset the timer and continue.

Once you are in motion, you may find it hard to stop. The activity builds a momentum that will probably carry you far beyond those first 5 minutes. It is not only possible, it's highly probable that you won't even *want* to stop.

This gimmick is rather like setting your wristwatch 5 minutes fast to keep from being late. It's deceptively simple, but it works.

Listless?

For those who just don't seem to know where to begin, making a "TO DO" list is helpful. A fresh list should be made each day.

If you generate too lengthy a list, you may be so overwhelmed all you can do is take two aspirin and a nap. Limit the list to the six most important things you have to accomplish. Set priorities on them. Start with the most important item and work it through to a conclusion. Then go on to number two.

If the same item shows up on your list day after day, you have a problem. You are procrastinating. Make the decision to *Do It Now* or cross it off your list. Either way you will be more productive.

CAUTION: Sometimes making a list gives you a false sense of accomplishment. A list is a plan, not a product.

Every couple of weeks review your lists to see if you are accomplishing anything of permanent value. It is easy to be so swamped with day-to-day activities that no constructive action is being taken toward some of your long-range goals. Remember, they are only goals if you are working toward them. Otherwise, they are merely dreams. Procrastinators are dreamers.

Do It Now!

Procrastinators have the habit of putting everything off until "later." To kick the habit, take action. *Do It Now!*

Put this book down! Get up and make that phone call, pay that bill, write that letter, clean that oven, enroll in that class, do those push-ups!

You may be a person haunted by a half-knitted afghan at the back of your closet. Everytime you handle it, you feel a sense of failure. "I *should* finish this afghan. I've been moving it around for 15 years." Give that almost-heirloom to a relative or donate it to Goodwill Industries. Get it out of your closet and into someone else's. You'll feel terrific.

Whenever possible take care of things that cross your desk (or your mind) right on the spot. If you don't, a stack of "stuff" will sprout and quickly engulf your desk, mantel, or dining room table. This stack usually consists of unanswered letters, bills, announcements, appeals, special offers, coupons, newspapers, magazines, receipts, and recipes.

Strive to handle each piece of paper only once. As you sort the daily mail, be decisive. Do you really want to subscribe to this magazine? Do you really want to contribute to this charity? Do you really want to read last Sunday's newspaper? If the answer to these questions is yes, *Do It Now*. If the answer is maybe, trash it. Adopt the motto: "If in doubt, throw it out!"

When you have an unpleasant task to perform, such as disciplining an employee, it is natural to want to avoid the task altogether. Accept the fact that some things are absolutely unavoidable. The longer you delay, the more you worry. As your anxiety increases, your ability to concentrate decreases. Your efficiency and effectiveness plummet.

Writing in *Getting Things Done: The ABC's of Time Management,* Edwin C. Bliss recommends starting each day by doing the most unpleasant thing on your "TO DO" list. Getting that thing out of the way first will make you feel exhilarated, almost euphoric. According to the author, an effective person approaches unpleasant tasks by saying, "This task is unpleasant, but it must be done; therefore I will do it now so I can forget about it."*

Go to Pieces

Because I love quilts so much, I used to wonder if I had the talent and perseverance to make one. Luckily, someone had invented a quilt-as-you-go method that allowed me to complete one little 12-inch block at a time. The grand plan was to finish twenty or thirty blocks and join them together to make a quilt.

Before I actually tried my hand at quilting, I aspired to making a queen-sized quilt. After struggling a few hours, I revised my goals and began thinking about a crib-sized quilt. I ended up making a pillow. One block was all I managed to complete.

I learned some valuable lessons from that experience: (1) you never know what you can (or can't) do until you actually try; (2) quilts can be bought; and (3) the key to accomplishing any large task is to break it down into little pieces. This applies to making a quilt, learning a new language, painting the house, cleaning the attic, writing a book, moving across country, or getting a college education.

College degrees, like quilts, can be pretty and practical or pretty impractical. It all depends on how they are made and how they are used.

If you are one of the many nurses who has been thinking about returning to school but are not sure you have the talent or perseverance required, try the learn-as-you-go method. Instead of letting the magnitude of the project overwhelm you, find a manageable piece.

Talk with a college advisor and have her spell out exactly what the college will require of you. Then take the college catalogue and read the course descriptions. Choose a course that not only meets college requirements but meets your personal requirements as well.

Choosing *one* class that looks interesting and has practical application in your real world will give you a sample of what it is like to be back in school. If you choose wisely, the class will be a satisfying

---

*Bliss, Edwin C.: Getting things done: the ABC's of time management, New York, 1976, Charles Scribner's Sons, p. 86.

experience in itself and also double as the first step toward a degree.

Committing yourself to a few weeks of classwork is less intimidating than committing to years of schooling. At any time you can revise your goals. After all, they are *your* goals.

On completing the first class, you may opt to take another, thus inching toward a degree. You may zealously decide to enroll full time. On the other hand, you may discover you do not want to be a student now or ever again. Working on your bachelor's degree can be crossed off your "TO DO" list. Redirect that time, energy, talent, and money toward something you really do want to do.

Time and Punishment

Behaviorists say that any activity followed by a reward is remembered pleasantly and tends to be repeated. Therefore, if you reward yourself for performing promptly, you will be on your way to breaking the procrastination habit.

Rewards may involve food, fun, friendship, or anything else you enjoy and usually indulge in each day. If you have a passion for coffee, you might decide to withhold coffee until you finish some appointed task. You allow yourself a cup of coffee only *after* you clean the closet, write Aunt Harriet, or finish your income tax forms. Until you complete your task, there will be no television, no phone calls, no luncheons, no shopping, or no bubble bath.

Some extremely stubborn procrastinators find the reward system needs to be enhanced by a punishment system. For example, if you fail to meet your deadline, you not only lose the reward, you enforce a punishment. You make yourself do something you hate—walk to work, take a cold shower, eat artichokes for breakfast, donate money to a political cause you oppose, or take a person you dislike to lunch.

Fear of Trying

There are many reasons why women may be more prone to procrastination than men. Little boys are encouraged to approach life in a rough-and-tumble manner. They are encouraged to "go for it!" Sure boys get hurt. That's part of life. But that's not supposed to be part of life for little girls.

Girls are cautioned to approach life in a safety-first manner. Just the thought of getting hurt is enough to deter girls from doing anything potentially dangerous. Unfortunately, anything potentially dangerous is also potentially fun and profitable.

Instead of wholeheartedly participating in life's scramble, girls sit on the sidelines. They grow up to be ladies-in-waiting, women who are not action oriented but reaction oriented. Programed to observe events and accept decisions, they pride themselves on their ability to respond, compromise, and accommodate.

The saying, "If life hands you a lemon, make lemonade," is descriptive of the way women are expected to handle life. Wait and see what life hands you, then do the best you can.

Goals can cause conflict for women because we have traditionally molded our lives around the goals of others. Once on the trail of our own goals, we are no longer as available as we once were. We are no longer as flexible. We can no longer be found cheering on the sidelines.

Sometimes that causes problems for other people like our husbands, children, parents, pastors, and employers. Since their problems have always been our problems, they may pressure us to postpone our own goals.

When you are feeling pressured, remember what management expert Peter F. Drucker says, "Most executives have learned that what one postpones, one actually abandons."*

Don't postpone or abandon your goals. Risk going after what you want. Don't wait for life to hand you a lemon, go out and pick what you really want.

If you just take life as it happens, you can always blame your misfortunes on luck or fate. Although that may dilute failure, it also waters down success because you can't take credit for your good fortune either.

Procrastinators are great believers in luck and fate.

Productive people have learned that future gain usually requires present pain. They have learned to risk, endure, sacrifice, and work *today,* so they can enjoy greater rewards tomorrow. Ask any successful dieter. Without pain there is no gain (or in the dieter's case, loss).

---

*Drucker, Peter F.: The effective executive, New York, 1967, Harper & Row, Publishers, Inc., p. 110.

It would be wonderful if women could learn to see risk as men do—a challenge, an opportunity, a win-some-lose-some proposition—and not be afraid to "go for it." Until we do, indecision and procrastination will continue to hamper us personally and professionally.

CHAPTER 9
Productivity

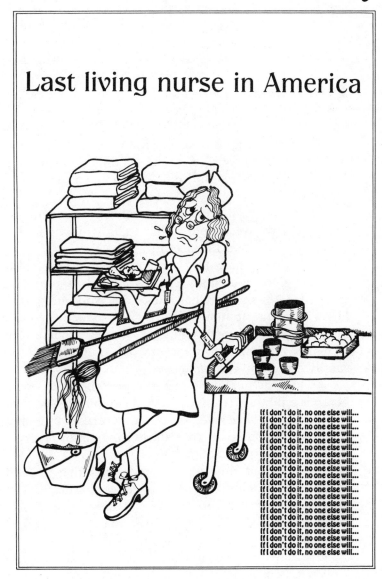

Last living nurse in America

For a moment let's forget all the flap about whether nursing is or is not a profession. Let's just roll up our sleeves and get down to business.

The formula for any successful business is to find a need and fill it—at a healthy profit, of course. Finding needs to fill isn't difficult. Need is everywhere. And nurses pride themselves on being "need-meeters."

Much like weed-eaters, which whirl around with lightning speed mowing down weeds, nurses like to mow down needs. "Show me a need, *any* need, and I'll meet it!"

As indiscriminate need-meeters, we whirl around taking care of everything for everybody everywhere. Remember the nurse who quipped, "Nursing is what nurses do. And nurses do everything!" His words sum up nursing's greatest productivity problem.

No one can do everything. Not even a nurse. Nurses have to recognize that although we are capable of doing almost *anything,* we simply cannot do *everything*.

As long as nursing remains vague about its own mission and goals, it can be easily distracted and exploited. Our reluctance to put a respectable dollar value on our time makes us a cheap, plentiful, and versatile source of labor subsidizing almost every other department in the hospital.

Much of our time is devoured facilitating the productivity of others. We've all been called on to cover pharmacy, take up the slack for dietary kitchen, transport patients to x-ray, act as security guards, make minor mechanical repairs, run to central supply, clean rooms, and deliver everything from mail to babies.

Occasionally such diverse chores are really nursing incognito. We straighten up a patient's room while we unobtrusively observe and interview. We transport seriously ill patients for their safety. We gather up dinner trays to keep better tabs on a particular patient's nutrition.

Most of the time, however, nurses do these chores because

"Somebody has to do it" or because "If I don't do it, no one else will." Those are direct quotes from indiscriminate need-meeters in action.

Deciding exactly what services nursing will provide is only half the battle. The other half is deciding what services nursing will *not* provide. Even nice nurses will have to learn to say no. We have to learn to be "discriminating need-meeters." We have to make conscious choices about *whose* needs we will meet, *which* needs we will meet, *where* we will meet those needs . . . *what* . . . *when* . . . *why* . . . and *how*.

Nurses are busy people, but being busy isn't the same as being productive. Busy or productive? It all depends on how we define:

The Business of Nursing

Productive people know how to mind their own business. Unfortunately, very few nurses have a clear idea of what their business is.

If I asked you to define the business of nursing in twenty-five words or less, what would *you* say? Go ahead, take a stab at it. I'll wait.

"As nurses our business is _____

_____

_____."

Chances are you skipped the above exercise dismissing the answer as either obvious or impossible. It is neither.

You may have searched your mind for cobwebbed remnants of those bio-psycho-social-cultural-spiritual-needing-wanting-life span definitions you memorized long ago. You may have come up with a definition similar to one of the following. Let me share some responses from other nurses who have tried to define the business of nursing.

What Is the Business of Nursing?

"Taking care of the sick"
"Alleviating the distress of patients by applying all our knowledge and expertise"

"To provide care for those who are ill and to prevent illness in those who are well"

"The giving of oneself for the care and benefit of others"

"Teaching patients to take care of themselves!"

"Seeing that the needs of a person are taken care of, either personally or through coordination with others—this includes all needs from physical to emotional to spiritual including family, friends, etc."

"The business of nursing is to do those things that are no one else's business."

"Dealing in health care, not only for the patient but for the family, from admission to discharge—either by physican or death"

"Caring"

"Taking care of patients' and physicians' problems, all of which require a lot of care"

"Providing a mutually agreeable service that assists clients to become functionally independent"

"Taking care of patients in all aspects using knowledge of good health care for both sick and well—it is a profession requiring lots of stamina, love, and knowledge."

"?????"

"Caring for human beings or educating them to care for themselves in an intelligent, efficient, and cost-effective manner"

"Charity—love and faith"

And my personal favorite from Ron Bayless, RN, poet laureate:

"Doing the necessary for the needy, being speedy, and not greedy."

You are bound to find some of the definitions appealing and some appalling. Each has its own merits. Each reflects choices made by the author. Collectively they serve to remind us that there is *no one right answer.*

Choice is the key. Of all the bio-psycho-social-*ad infinitum* needs waiting to be met, nursing has yet to make a conscious, deliberate, and courageous choice.

Examining nursing as a business and not as a duty, calling, or profession may be novel enough to bring new insights to some old problems that have plagued us for years. Although I don't have all the answers, I think I have identified the most important question to ask of nursing today: "What is our business?"

Where do we begin to find an answer to that question? The root of any business definition is the customer. The customer is the *only* reason for any business to exist. It is the customer's wants, wishes, needs, and values that guide the business.

Who is nursing's customer? *The Patient.*

That answer is not wrong, but it is not right either. The patient is just *one* of nursing's customers. Actually very few patients engage nurses directly in a buyer-seller-of-service transaction. Most nurses wholesale themselves to an employer—hospital, doctor, clinic, school, agency. The employer then sells a complex package of products and services to the customer, which includes nursing care.

Who is another of nursing's customers? *The Employer.*

Once nursing wholesales itself to an employer, it loses much control over its practice and utilization. In a sense, the employer "owns" nursing. Bought and paid for, nursing must then bend to the employer's decisions on utilization, practice, deployment, direction, and appropriation.

Nurses are not the only professionals who wholesale themselves. Any doctor or lawyer who gives up private practice for a salaried position must regard the employer as a most important customer.

Nurses who have been taught to focus almost exclusively on the patient and encouraged to strive for professional autonomy are bound to be confused and frustrated by the realities of employment. Our educational background leaves us woefully ignorant of politics, economics, management, and organizational behavior.

Speaking of our educational background, perhaps many of the disputes between nursing education and nursing service would evaporate if education looked upon service as its prime customer. For years nursing service has objected to new graduates who are all thumbs and theory. Nursing education simply is not listening to its customer.

The only way to increase our productivity is to know what we are to produce. The only way to know what to produce is to scrutinize our customers—all our customers. We have to know who they are, where they are, and what they want or need or value enough to actually purchase.

An initial description of nursing's customers might be condensed to read:

Who are our customers?	*Everyone*
Where are our customers?	*Everywhere*
What do they value?	*Everything*

When pressed for more details, nurses have produced lists like these:

WHO ARE OUR CUSTOMERS?	WHERE ARE OUR CUSTOMERS?
Patients	In hospitals
Doctors	In waiting rooms
Hospitals	In clinics
Schools	At the health department
Communities	Factories
Government	Schools
Families	Churches
Ill-well–young-old	On the telephone
Industry	In the streets
Nursing service	At home
All creatures great and small	From nurseries to nursing homes

WHAT DO OUR CUSTOMERS VALUE?

Comfort!	Being normal	Efficiency
Independence	Their life	Effectiveness
Mobility	Speedy recovery	Anticipation of needs
Health	Knowledge	Individualized attention
Money	Respect	Expert opinion
Themselves	Privacy	Compassion
Traditions	Nurturance	Dignity
Quality care	Politeness	Not enough!
	Promptness	

Keeping these lists in mind, let's zero in on a few of those what-is-the-business-of-nursing definitions and see what implications they might have if chosen by nursing as its business definition.

The business of nursing is "taking care of the sick."

A wellness buff would have a minor stroke after reading the above definition. But before judging the author too harshly, consider one thing: her definition makes nursing manageable. She does not see nursing as a do-everything-for-everybody-everywhere profession. Like Kentucky Fried Chicken, she wants to "do one thing and do it right!" That formula has worked well for physicians. They do a good job of meeting a very few specific needs. Some worry that indeed their services are too few and too specific.

Concerned that doctors' almost single-minded focus on the biological basis of illness was inhibiting their ability to help patients, Dr. Daniel Silverman, Director of Outpatient Psychiatry at Beth Israel in Boston, undertook a study.* Using Harvard Medical School students, he created a course emphasizing the psychosocial aspects of illness.

Even after a semester of concentrated exposure to such concepts as personality, life-style, and job-related stress in addition to special tutoring by psychiatrists, medical students still showed a "biological bias." At the beginning, middle, and end of the course (which offered no instruction concerning tests and procedures), the students were shown videotapes of simulated medical interviews. They were then asked to list, in order of importance, other kinds of information they would want before prescribing treatment.

Ninety percent of the requests were for lab tests and other biological information. Practicing doctors at Beth Israel who were shown the same videotapes responded with an even greater biological orientation.

Doctors know their business. They fill *a* need. They do not feel compelled to meet *all* needs. They specialize and make a healthy profit by knowing more and more about less and less.

The business of nursing is "to provide care for those who are ill and to prevent illness in those who are well."

This two-pronged approach is more ambitious and less manageable than just "taking care of the sick." It forces us to divide nursing resources (time, energy, education, personnel) allocating some to care for the sick and others to keep people well.

Most nurses spend their professional lives taking care of the sick. The need is obvious. The money is there. It's tradition!

But traditions are being broken by health maintenance organizations that profit when people are well, not when they are sick. Many industrial giants like General Electric are launching programs to cut their health bills by encouraging healthier life-styles for their em-

---

*Silverman, D., et al.: In search of the biopsychosocial perspective: an experiment with beginning medical students, Am. J. Psychiatry **140**(9):1154-1159, 1983.

ployees, retirees, and dependents. GE is sponsoring health fairs, screening for high blood pressure and glaucoma, and using computers to find the best prices among hospitals and physicians.

The business of nursing is "giving oneself for the care and benefit of others."

When *RN* magazine in their September 1983 issue reported on what a nurse means when she says, "I'm a professional," one nurse wrote that the true professional "serves others without regard for monetary compensation."★ By that standard, nurses may be the only "true professionals."

"Giving oneself" speaks of sacrifice, not success. Once again we see a nurse's confusion between career and charity. We see the difficulty many have when it comes to even discussing nursing as a business.

CAUTION, NURSES: Nothing given away is ever appreciated. If you do not place a high value on your time, talent, education, experience, and ability, no one else will either.

Like it or not, in our society the pervading feeling is that as the price increases, so does the value of the service or product.

Designer jeans—same denim, same thread, same fit, same wear. Add a designer's name and double the price.

Health care—same goal, same approach, same information, same treatment. Add a doctor's name and double the price.

People seeking "professional" care expect to pay for it. If they do not have to pay for it, they regard it as unprofessional.

The business of nursing is "seeing that the needs of a person are taken care of, either personally or through coordination with others. This includes all needs from physical to emotional to spiritual including family, friends, etc."

Beware the "et cetera."

One of the most scathing reviews of an actor was that "he suffered from delusions of adequacy." Every time I hear nurses exhorted to meet *all* needs physical, emotional, and spiritual, I wonder if nurses aren't suffering from "delusions of adequacy."

★Gulack, R.: What a nurse means when she says "I'm a professional," RN **46:**29, Sept. 1983.

By refusing to put boundaries on the scope of nursing, we set ourselves up for much frustration and ultimate failure. One nurse and one profession cannot be all things to all people.

The business of nursing is "to do those things that are no one else's business."

I love this definition. When we are asked what nurses do, it enables us to say, "None of your business!"

Actually, it is very descriptive. For years nurses have followed doctors through the health care field, like gleaners, picking up the leftovers. (You may recall in biblical times gleaning was an acceptable way to survive. After the landowners had harveted a field, gleaners went through gathering up grain left behind.)

Nurses often behave as if doctors owned the health care field and were generous to let nurses pick up anything they didn't want. Come to think of it, doctors often behave that way too.

Today a multitude of health care specialists have joined doctors tramping through the field. Unlike nurses, each group seems to know exactly what it wants to reap.

Nurses continue to trail behind trying to sustain the profession on leftovers. Many feel our meager existence is threatened.

Gleaners may survive, but they never thrive. Many nurses, tired of gleaning, leave the health care field altogether. Others decide to get up a little earlier in the morning and beat some of those Johnny-come-latelies into the field. Some have actually bought their own fields.

If you find you're in the wrong field, even for the right reasons, you may not survive. If your field is full of weeds, overworked, eroded, or nonproductive, perhaps it is time to change fields. Heaven knows the whole field of wellness seems up for grabs.

The business of nursing is "?????"

For many of us nursing has been reduced to a series of question marks. Is nursing a profession? A job? A career? An art? A science? A dependent, independent, or interdependent activity?

Much like a centipede pondering which foot to put down first, nursing sits immobilized by indecision. Our theorists, philosophers, and leaders need to stop pondering and put a foot down—any foot. It's always better to be limping than paralyzed.

Perhaps you and I can put things in motion by making some decisions of our own. Even though we might not presume to speak for "the profession" or for "the hospital," we might be able to speak for our individual units or departments.

Consider one business definition of nursing that we haven't yet explored. It is simply "caring." Perhaps this single word best encompasses nursing.

If you look up care and caring in the dictionary, you will find this descriptive phrase: "a disquieted state of blended uncertainty, apprehension, and responsibility." (If that's not synonymous with nursing, what is?)

Another phrase used in the definition of caring is "painstaking or watchful attention." Watchful attention—that's why people submit to hospitalization. They need watchful attention.

Painstaking or watchful attention is the very core of nursing. When attention ceases, caring ceases. Nursing ceases. It doesn't matter whether inattention is a result of fatigue, absence, indifference, or ignorance. The result is the same.

If you were to ask your coworkers, "What is our business here on 5-West?" they might think you daffy because the answer is so obvious. "Why caring for patients, of course!" they would reply. "Caring is our business."

Caring is a one-word business definition that says everything or nothing depending on how it is applied. Taking caring from the abstract and putting it into action is a highly complex task.

There is one unit that has accomplished that task elegantly. It is an inpatient oncology unit at the University Hospital in Madison, Wisconsin.

Two clinical nurse specialists, Ann Paulen and Catherine Rapp, in essence asked, "What is our business on this unit?" Their answer was "Person-Centered Caring."* They proceeded to write standards and operational guidelines that made it possible to convert lofty philosophical concepts into practical actions.

---

*Paulen, Ann, and Rapp, Catherine: Person-centered caring, Nurs. Manage. **12**:17, Sept. 1981.

Standards for person-centered caring*

I. Humanness
  A. Standard
    The patient's and family's humanness is respected.
  B. Outcome criteria
    The patient and family state that:
    1. They are treated like human beings
    2. They are addressed by their preferred names
    3. Their values and life style are respected
    4. Their rights are upheld
  C. Process criteria
    The nurse will:
    1. Assess patient/family values and/or life style
    2. Use the name(s) the patient/family prefer
    3. Encourage patient's personalization of environment
    4. Uphold patient/family rights
II. Family†
  A. Standard
    The patient and family are treated as a unit.
  B. Outcome criteria
    The patient and family state that:
    1. Their relationship is respected
    2. They participate in care as desired
    3. They have the information they want/need
  C. Process criteria
    The nurse will:
    1. Appreciate the effect of one member's illness on the family unit
    2. Counsel/teach/include the family as well as the patient
III. Rights
  A. Standard
    The patient's and family's rights are upheld.
  B. Outcome criteria
    The patient and family state that:
    1. They are treated like human beings
    2. They receive the information they want
    3. They are involved in decision making to the extent desired

---

*Paulen, Ann, and Rapp, Catherine: Person-centered caring, Nurs. Manage. **12:**17, Sept. 1981. By permission.
†Family is defined as a social unit which includes significant friends as well as immediate and extended family.

4. They are supported when either accepting or rejecting treatment plans/recommendations
5. They are comfortable with confidentiality of personal information
6. Their privacy is considered
7. Resources desired are made available to them

C. Process criteria

The nurse will:

1. Discuss the patient's/family's rights with them
2. Act as an advocate for the patient/family
3. Assess information/education needs with the patient/family
4. Provide information/education for the patient/family
5. Involve the patient/family in decision making as they desire
6. Provide for patient/family privacy
7. Ensure confidentiality of information
8. Facilitate access to interdisciplinary resources

IV. Coping

A. Standard

The patient's and family's coping skills are respected.

B. Outcome criteria

The patient and family state that:

1. Their adaptation to health/illness is respected
2. The opportunity for expanding coping skills is offered
3. Their use of support systems is facilitated

C. Process criteria

The nurse will:

1. Respect patient/family coping skills
2. Offer the opportunity for learning alternative coping skills
3. Facilitate the use of patient/family support systems

V. Choice

A. Standard

Patients' control over their life and death is facilitated.

B. Outcome criteria

Patients state that:

1. They are treated as partners in their health care
2. They have sufficient information for decision making
3. Their right to informed choice is protected
4. Their suggestions for modifying physical and emotional comfort are sought and considered

C. Process criteria
   The nurse will:
   1. Treat patients as partners in their health care
   2. Protect the patient's right to informed choice
   3. Act as an advocate for patients
   4. Seek patient/family input in planning and evaluating symptom management

VI. Continuity
   A. Standard
      Continuity of caring is fostered.
   B. Outcome criteria
      The patient and family state that:
      1. Ongoing health/illness care is compatible with their values and life style
      2. They have the information and resources needed for continuing health care
      3. They are developing adequate relationships with member(s) of the health care system
      4. They know whom to contact with questions/concerns
   C. Process criteria
      The nurse will:
      1. Collaborate with the patient/family to individualize continuing health/illness care
      2. Plan for ongoing followup (including bereavement counseling)
      3. Facilitate access to community resources

They did much more than write standards and file them away to gather dust. They made these standards part of the day-to-day functioning of their unit.

To see if person-centered caring is attained, patients and their families are interviewed. The standards are also used in nurse interviews and incorporated in yearly evaluation conferences. Periodically charts and care plans are pulled at random and checked to see if all these good intentions are in actual operation and well documented.

For example, staff nurse interviews include questions like: "Do you treat patients as partners in their health care? How do you do this? Do you involve patients and their families in care and decision making as they desire? What do you include when discussing patients' rights? How do you consider patient and family values and life-style? Do you treat patients like human beings?"

Some patient interview questions include: "Are you as involved in decisions about your health care as you want to be? Do you feel the staff respects the way you are responding to your illness and hospitalization? Are you satisfied with the way your family and friends are treated? Are you called by the name you prefer? Do you feel you are being treated like a human being by the staff?"

That last question is difficult for nurses to ask. It is not difficult for patients to answer.

Paulen and Rapp have found that most patients don't expect much more than safe physical care and common courtesy. They are utterly surprised and delighted when treated as humans with rights and choices.

Nurses are also humans with rights and choices. Even if you cannot speak for the profession, the hospital, or the unit, you can speak for yourself.

"As a nurse, my business is _____

_____

_____ ."

One nurse wrote the business of nursing is "teaching patients to take care of themselves!" Although she may not be able to convince her profession, employer, or even co-workers to adopt this definition, she can choose to adopt it.

Once her mission becomes teaching patients to care for themselves, her goals are much clearer. Patient teaching is her top priority. She can no longer relegate it to those few chance moments between her "real" nursing chores.

Working for an employer who does not share her values will be counterproductive at best. This nurse will be most satisfied and satisfactory working in areas that promote preventive medicine or focus on patient self-care. She might find a patient educator position most appealing.

If she decides to pursue a degree, her course work will have to reflect her values and priorities if it is to be at all meaningful or productive.

To be most productive she may actually have to leave the hospital. She might be better utilized in public health or as an industrial consultant. If she has an entrepreneurial spirit, she might go into business for herself helping people to stop smoking, control their weight, or manage stress. For a person with this business definition, these are all legitimate extensions of nursing.

Until we nurses decide collectively, locally, and individually just what our business is, we cannot increase our productivity.

The choice is ours: caring for the sick . . . keeping people well . . . doing what we are told . . . teaching patients self-care . . . facilitating the work of other professionals. . . .

The decisions we make will shape our educational policies, set our professional standards, guide our daily work, and ultimately determine our future.

Listen to one last nurse's response to "What is the business of Nursing?":

> I would like to answer this question with my *only* answer: "Nursing *is* my business. For the past 27 years it has provided me with an excellent income and been most rewarding in every phase."

Nursing is *my* business too. Let's mind our own business.

CHAPTER 10

Professional Rights and Responsibilities

Exercise your rights!

The right to:

- Be treated with respect
- A reasonable workload
- An equitable wage
- Set your own priorities
- Ask for what you want
- Refuse without making excuses or feeling guilty
- Make mistakes and be responsible for them
- Give and receive information as a professional
- Act in the best interest of the patient
- Be human

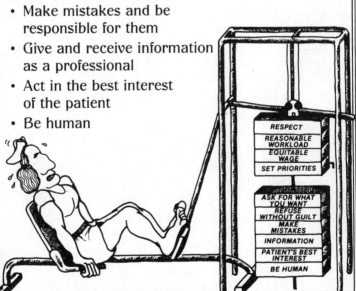

R ounding a curve on the coastal highway, I spot a rain-drenched hitchhiker. He raises his thumb and smiles hopefully at me.

Chances are he's a poet, a free spirit, or a wandering student who's out to experience life. But there is also a chance that he's a psychotic, a thief, or a murderer. At 50 mph I can't distinguish poets from psychotics, so I don't take chances.

I zip past him and my spirits are briefly dampened by feelings of guilt. *Guilt* . . . because I was reared and educated to be a helper . . . because I was taught to share . . . because I believe in being a Good Samaritan . . . because I'm a "have" and he's a "have not."

I am drawn to a need like a moth to a flame. Unlike the moth, however, I know I can get burned. I *know* better than to pick up hitchhikers. Yet, in that split second our eyes meet, I *feel* compelled to help him. I have to consciously resist the urge to stop.

Why do I feel responsible for every stray living being on life's highway? Because I am a responsible person. It's as automatic as the knee-jerk reflex. When I perceive a person has a need or a right, I feel a responsibility. Your right—my responsibility.

No wonder people take advantage of me!

My problem lies in my misinterpretation of people's needs and rights. They are not synonymous. The hitchhiker needs a ride. He has a right to thumb a ride. He does not have a right to a ride.

My responsibility stops at respecting his right to hitchhike. I am not responsible for his transportation.

You have a right to freedom of speech. I respect your right. I have no responsibility to listen to you.

In a very real sense, your rights are also your responsibilities. You have the right to free speech, but it is *your* responsibility to attract and hold an audience.

I *could* give the hitchhiker a ride. I *could* listen to you. Should I? That's the question that haunts responsible people.

Nurses are responsible people. We have dwelled so long and so hard on our responsibilities, we are often surprised at the prospect of having rights ourselves. Rights always seem to belong to other people. Perhaps that's why Ten Basic Rights for Women in the Health Professions is the most frequently requested reprint from *STAT*.*

To refresh your memory, here are those basic rights:

1. You have the right to be treated with respect.
2. You have the right to a reasonable work load.
3. You have the right to an equitable wage.
4. You have the right to determine your own priorities.
5. You have the right to ask for what you want.
6. You have the right to refuse without making excuses or feeling guilty.
7. You have the right to make mistakes and be responsible for them.
8. You have the right to give and receive information as a professional.
9. You have the right to act in the best interest of the patient.
10. You have the right to be human.

These rights are yours, but acquiring and holding them is *your* responsibility. Not the doctor's. Not the head nurse's. Not the administrator's. Yours.

Let's revisit each of these ten rights and see some of the dilemmas and delights they pose for responsible people:

You Have the Right to be Treated with Respect

Mutual respect is absolutely essential if there is to be any semblance of a health care *team*. Unfortunately, I am inundated with examples of doctor-nurse interactions in which respect is sorely lacking.

Doctors often behave as if they had a right to humiliate nurses. Nurses often behave as if they had a responsibility to stand there and be humiliated.

> On many occasions while working as an RN/Scrub Assistant we were told that "even a goddamn monkey can be taught to scrub." We were referred to at various times as stupid and slow. My only response was to pout and throw icy stares. (Very effective. Ha ha!)

---

*Chenevert, Melodie: STAT: special techniques in assertiveness training for women in the health professions, St. Louis, 1983, The C.V. Mosby Co.

As long as nurses submit to such humiliation, it will continue. Pouts and icy stares are not effective deterrents because they are too easily ignored. You can get the surgeon's attention by clamping a hemostat on his nose or handing him the wrong end of a scalpel, but those actions tend to escalate hostilities, not increase mutual respect.

Any team tortured and humiliated by its "captain" is not a winning team. If you believe teamwork is in the best interest of your patients, you must confront the surgeon.

Give him the phone number of the zoo and walk out. Nurses are not in the monkey business. Either the insulting behavior is discontinued, or the doctor works alone.

It can be done. Here's proof.

One OR supervisor tells of an irascible doctor who had alienated every scrub nurse on her staff with his haughty demeanor, sarcastic speech, and innumerable temper tantrums. At length every veteran scrub nurse absolutely refused to work with him.

A brand-new nurse had just joined the staff, and it was her luckless lot to be assigned to the beast. Within moments he had reduced her to tears. He stormed out of the room and confronted the supervisor. How dare she assign him some bumbling novice!

The supervisor stood toe-to-toe and eye-to-eye with the surgeon and said calmly, "Doctor, there is not a single nurse on my staff who will scrub with you. That new nurse is your last chance. If she won't assist you, no one will." She pivoted and walked away.

Once out of sight, she ducked into the nearest broom closet. Her knees were like jelly, and her heart was beating so fast she thought she would collapse.

The surgeon paused, then reentered the operating room. He proceeded to make the novice into a first-rate colleague. They are still a splendid team.

Another physician was famous for throwing patients' charts when he became irritated. One day he threw a chart, splattering its contents all over the end of the hall.

The nurse who was accompanying him on rounds immediately knelt to pick it up. From afar the head nurse bellowed, **"Don't pick up that chart!"** The nurse froze. In a quieter tone the head nurse continued, "The doctor dropped the chart, the doctor will pick it up."

The doctor stared at the head nurse in disbelief. Then he stepped over the chart and stomped off the floor.

An hour later he returned and asked for Mrs. So-and-So's chart. The head nurse replied, "It's at the end of the hall where you left it." The doctor retrieved it. He has never thrown another chart—at least not on that floor.

If nurses are to gain respect, we must behave in a "respectable" manner. Respect must be earned. Groveling, cowering, and kowtowing are not actions that command respect.

You Have the Right to a Reasonable Work Load

As a new graduate, I was a head nurse. It was a small unit—10 beds. My "staff" consisted of me and an aide. I was responsible for medications, treatments, charting, rounds with physicians, direct patient care, etc.

I consistently worked overtime and asked to be paid for it. The director of nurses repeatedly stated there was no reason for the overtime, and I shouldn't have to be paid.

Finally, in response to her constant harassment, I only asked to be paid overtime occasionally. Often I went home in tears still feeling I deserved to be paid for what I was doing.

The terms *new graduate* and *head nurse* should be mutually exclusive. They should never be synonymous.

Not only is this new graduate in water over her head, she is going down for the third time. Hearing her cries for help, the director of nurses scolds her for drowning. Instead of throwing a life preserver, she throws stones.

Overtime is not the problem. It is a symptom of the problem. Whether the problem lies within the new nurse or within the hospital system, nothing is being done to correct it.

The young nurse will not be with that hospital long. With this sort of initiation into nursing, she won't be in the profession long. As for the director of nursing, well . . . she obviously lacks organizational management skills every bit as much as the new graduate.

A clinical nurse specialist was hired to spend 30 percent of her time with the perinatal team. At weekly "team" meetings she was constantly harassed by the physicians who demanded she explain why she was not doing everything a full-time person could do.

She tried reasoning with them. She explained that 30 percent of a 40 hour week is only 12 hours. One person can only do so much in that short amount of time. But the doctors continued to push and complain.

The meetings exhausted her. Afterward, feeling humiliated and defeated, she retreated to her office to lick her wounds. She began to dread those meetings so much she was thinking of resigning.

Then at an assertiveness workshop she learned a new technique called fogging. That's a comical name for a very effective technique. During verbal attacks you stand calmly sifting through the barrage for a small statement that has a bit of truth to it. When the attack subsides, you agree with the tiny truth, and then make your counter-proposal.

At the next meeting she sat calmly through the doctors' criticism. Then she looked at them and said, "Gentlemen, you are absolutely right. You do need a clinical nurse specialist full-time. I am prepared to leave the hospital staff and come to work for you directly. For $25,000 a year you can have my undivided attention."

The doctors were speechless. It never occurred to them that if they wanted more service, they would have to pay for it.

In subsequent meetings, if a criticism arose, the nurse just reiterated her offer and smiled.

> I am a nurse administrator in a medical/surgical/psychiatric setting. I am required to function both as a team leader and nursing supervisor.
>
> Recently our part-time psychiatrist who was responsible for the 90-day reviews of patient progress and revision of psychiatric treatment plans resigned. The administration informed me that I would assume this responsibility.
>
> I objected, especially since this would not include a salary raise. I must not have been assertive enough because I was coerced into doing this.

This nurse is one of the multitude of nurses employed by institutions that are generous with responsibilities and stingy with rewards and recognition. Hospitals don't expect nurses to negotiate. They expect them to do as they are told.

And we do!

A skilled, self-respecting professional would negotiate a fee for service or a contract comparable to the one enjoyed by the part-time psychiatrist. Actually, a nurse could probably provide quality service at half the cost and save the hospital a bundle while making herself a fortune. That should make everyone happy. Unfortunately, this nurse works at Ebenezer Scrooge Memorial. They don't want to pay less. They want to pay nothing.

Perhaps this nurse can function adequately as a pseudopsychiatrist. Does the Board of Nursing think so? What about the JCAH? These factors enter into any negotiation.

If salary cannot be negotiated, work load must. Before picking up this new responsibility, negotiate exactly what will be put down. Few nurses have the time necessary to absorb such a large and important task. Being team leader and supervisor is bound to keep this nurse busy. If she is to be their "psychiatrist," which do they want to relieve her of: team leading or supervising?

Her last comment about being "coerced into doing this" could be echoed by every overworked nurse. How did they coerce her? Did they chain her to a desk and withhold food and water until she completed those 90-day reviews? Did they beat her? Did they hold her family hostage?

No. They sang a few choruses of the "If-You-Don't-Do-It-No-One-Else-Will Blues." They implied the patients would suffer if she did not do as she was told. They called her sense of duty, loyalty, and professionalism into question. They threatened her with the loss of her "nice-nurse" reputation.

She was not coerced. She was flimflammed.

You Have the Right to an Equitable Wage

After speaking at a national conference, I was taken aside by a woman who objected to my use of the term *wage*. As a nursing instructor she taught her students that "workers earn wages, professionals earn salaries."

Considering the fact that many nurses are required to punch time clocks and are often paid less than unskilled male laborers, I think I'll stick with the word wage.

> I have been employed at "St. Ignats" for 9 years. My job title is nursing practitioner. My job responsibilities presently include direct clinical service, staff and student nurse supervision, and program planning. In the past I have had administrative responsibilities and directed staff in-service. I have wanted to upgrade my position for a long time.
>
> About 5 years ago I half-heartedly talked with the director of staffing and recruitment for nursing, stating that I had many more

responsibilities than the average staff nurse. I allowed myself to be put off by her reasoning that as the only nurse in my department I would be unable to get a higher position regardless of my responsibilities. I have not spoken with her again about this matter. I would like to try again and this time succeed.

Isn't it amazing how easily nurses are controlled by any statement masquerading as logic. I can hear the director cooing, "Yes, I know you have many more responsibilities than the average staff nurse. But you are the only nurse in your department. You are already at the top. There is no way you can be given a higher position."

Why wouldn't the director's reasoning apply to the head of General Motors or the administrator of the hospital? Because it is not logical. Their salaries reflect the responsibilities they assume. As responsibilities increase, so do reward and recognition—except in nursing.

This director is a master of managerial politics. I know because I was once asked to speak at a conference by that title, and whenever I am asked to speak, I consult a dictionary to look up all the words in the conference theme or title. (I hope people conducting conferences do the same.)

Preparing for that particular conference, I looked up managerial politics in my dictionary and explored all ramifications of those two words. I assembled many possible meanings for the phrase. My favorite was "to make and keep submissive by artful and often dishonest practices." Although I am sure the conference organizers did not have that particular combination in mind, that definition captures the director's behavior.

For years this rather exploited nurse has shouldered her share of responsibilities. Now she wants more. She wants the rewards and recognition that should accompany her position. Unlike the head of General Motors and the hospital administrator, however, she is not sure she "deserves" them.

Her lack of confidence in her own worth defeated her 5 years ago when she "half-heartedly" approached the director. Lack of confidence will defeat her again. Salaries, like respect, have to be earned. You have to command them.

After 15 years as a part-time float nurse in a 250 bed hospital, I was offered the position of relief supervisor from 4 PM to midnight.

I was given a 50 cent an hour raise and promised I would be reviewed in 6 months.

Six months passed—no review.
Twelve months passed—no review.
Eighteen months passed—no review.

The director of nursing had multiple personal problems during this time, so I kept making excuses for her delay. But after 18 months, I made an appointment to see her about it.

She said my review had completely skipped her mind. Then, because I was already making "top staff-nurse wages," she wasn't sure a raise was in order. She promised to think about it.

Two weeks later she called me in and offered me a 6-cent raise. Yes! Six cents!!! After performing as a supervisor for a year and a half, she offered me a 6-cent raise.

I resigned my supervisory position at that meeting and returned to being a float nurse. It was one of the most difficult things I have ever done.

Six months later she called me in and offered me $3 an hour over top staff-nurse wages if I would become supervisor again. I happily agreed. I love being a supervisor.

I consider that 6 months I went back to floating the most valuable 6 months of my career. I have to say those were also the hardest 6 months of my life.

Was it worth it? You bet it was!

You Have the Right to Determine Your Own Priorities

If you don't exercise your right to set your own priorities, you will get plenty of exercise attending to other people's priorities.

I wish I had been more assertive when I took my present job—combined clinical and classroom teaching:

Too much work
Too little pay
Too little time to prepare lectures, grade papers, counsel students, meetings, etc.

I like my job, but it's too much to handle, especially when we are expected to get a masters on our own time. I have a husband and young son at home. I feel exhausted much of the work year.

115

This nurse is caught in the cross fire of competing priorities. She can't keep everyone happy. Her best bet is to set and honor her own priorities, or she will be pulled apart by other people's unrealistic demands. She needs to accept the fact that other people's priorities are not necessarily her priorities.

Her plight reminds me of a newlywed nurse who used to rise quietly so she wouldn't wake her sleeping husband and tiptoe around the house getting ready for work. When she left at 6:15 AM, he was still sleeping peacefully. He didn't have to leave for work for a full 2 hours.

Arriving home in the late afternoon, she dashed madly about cleaning and cooking. When her husband arrived home, he dropped into his favorite chair, read the paper, and relaxed. After dinner their evenings were free for romance. Ah, youth!

The young husband never once washed the dishes or performed any other household chore. It never occurred to either of them that he should.

More than a year passed. The nurse found she was too tired for romantic evenings. She fell asleep soon after dinner. In the early morning hours, she began to resent her sleeping husband as she hurriedly dressed for work.

Then one day her husband called it to her attention that a colleague's wife got up at 5:00 AM so she could wax the floors before leaving for work. He added, "Maybe you ought to try that."

Something snapped. From that moment on the days of the marriage were numbered.

When the nurse married again, her priorities had changed substantially. She chose a husband who would share the work as well as the fun. They've been happily married almost 20 years.

Passions cool. Priorities change. Important things on one day may be insignificant the next. Just remember, there are no wrong priorities as long as they're *your* priorities.

You Have the Right to Ask for What You Want

This is one right I have considered rephrasing. Nurses are so hesitant to ask for what they *need,* they cannot accept the idea of asking for what they want. It seems too self-indulgent.

For example, a recently widowed nurse with young children found her full-time job and single-parent responsibilities overwhelming. She wanted to reduce her work week to 4 days. Although she could manage on the reduced salary, having a handicapped child made a concurrent reduction in health care coverage unbearable.

For weeks she agonized over her dilemma. Finally she screwed up her courage and made an appointment with the administrator. Preparing for that appointment, she gathered facts, figures, and testimonials. She rehearsed responses to any questions or arguments he might have.

Once in his office she began, "I can only work 4 days a week, but I simply must have full health coverage."

Before she could continue, he said, "Fine."

"What?"

"I said that's fine."

She thanked him and nearly danced out of the office. She kicked herself for not having asked sooner.

Another nurse writes:

> As a part-time relief nurse, I was being sent to every unit in the hospital. The chief of nursing, being an ex-army nurse, felt that *any* nurse should be able to work *any* place needed in the hospital.
>
> One evening she ordered me to go to the emergency room. I went to her office and refused saying I wasn't knowledgeable or experienced enough to work in that area. She agreed and sent me elsewhere. What a relief!

Happy endings—they are never guaranteed, but you will rarely get what you want unless you ask for it.

You Have the Right to Refuse Without Making Excuses or Feeling Guilty

Whenever a nurse refuses a request or a command from a superior, she feels guilty. She feels guilty even if she is within her rights, even if it is her responsibility to refuse.

Here are two examples in which nurses refused. Backed by knowledge, experience, and hospital policy, they held their ground. They were not comfortable, but they refused to be intimidated.

> As weekend charge nurse, I was ordered to give uncross-matched blood, but no physician would sign to take responsibility in case of a reaction. I was told to sign—"everything will be

117

okay"—yet not one of the three doctors involved would sign themselves.

Firmly I told the doctors, "No signature. No blood." Later I received an apology and a thanks.

The following nurse is caught in a crunch between a hospital policy and a physician who thinks he is above such policies.

Several weeks ago I received a lab result of a fasting blood sugar of 675 on a diabetic patient who was on insulin. I called the patient's MD who told me to call the patient and tell him to change his insulin dosage.

Hospital policy states we cannot take telephone orders. I informed the MD of this. He became very nasty on the phone stating nurses were stupid and had stupid rules, etc. About a half hour later he came to the clinic and started to write the order for the insulin increase. Suddenly he decided the patient should be admitted and changed the orders. While there he again made insulting remarks about nurses.

The patient was called and advised to come to the hospital. He remained in the hospital 3 weeks.

I felt despite the MD's insulting and abusive remarks I had asserted my rights as a nurse and an individual.

It is far better to refuse than capitulate and risk a serious error. Failure to refuse can make you a sorry excuse for a nurse.

You Have the Right to Make Mistakes and Be Responsible for Them

Not surprisingly, it is difficult to get workshop participants to share examples of mistakes they have made. Professionals don't make mistakes. I wish that were true.

Although being a professional lessens the chance of error, it does not eliminate the possibility of mistakes. Acknowledging our mistakes is painful but necessary for professional growth.

When I was working a night shift, I had an LPN, another RN, and an older aide working with me. One night a patient fell and was unconscious on the floor.

I told everybody not to move the patient and started to take vital signs. The older aide said, "We have to move him to bed because we can't have a code on the floor." She started moving him with the LPN's help.

When the doctor came in and saw the patient, he said we should not have moved him because of the possibility of a cervical fracture. And I felt bad.

The nurse in this situation made a grave error. Her mistake was caused by lack of confidence in her own professional judgment. She allowed an aide to usurp her authority. If the patient is injured, it is the nurse, not the aide, who must accept the responsibility.

The incident is symptomatic of a much larger problem. Not only does this nurse need to review basic first aid, she needs to gain the skill and confidence necessary to effectively exert the authority of her position and her profession. Sometimes I think we need a nationwide confidence-building program for nurses.

You Have the Right to Give and Receive Information as a Professional

Nurses have both the right and the responsibility of keeping doctors informed about their patients. Yet many nurses dread telephoning physicians because they have received so many tongue lashings. Here's how one nurse solved the problem:

> A doctor was yelling over the phone, using abusive language, saying nothing really pertinent to this patient's care.
>
> Amid the yelling I said, "I can see you're upset. I'm going to hang up the phone and call you back in 5 minutes. I hope we can discuss your patient's problem calmly.

She hung up. Five minutes later she called him back. Their conversation was polite and productive.

> I'm a public health nurse. When visiting an elderly gentleman who was bedridden and cared for totally by his wife, I found he had rales in his lungs, a temperature, and irregular respirations.
>
> I phoned his doctor who said, "Well, what do you expect me to do about it? He's dying!"
>
> I said, "What you do about it is your responsibility. But it is my responsibility to inform you of changes in the patient's condition."
>
> His tone mellowed and he offered to visit the gentleman at home. I was in shock. Assertiveness could be a dangerous thing for me to know!

The public health nurse exercised her right in a very responsible manner.

You Have the Right to Act in the Best Interest of the Patient

Often nurses have to act in the best interest of their patients because the patients cannot speak for themselves.

> I work as a staff nurse in a hospital OB nursery. One of the baby's bilirubin tests was quite high, and I was anxious to report this to the doctor so treatment could be started.
>
> Well, the doctor arrived and did nothing about this situation. I knew this was wrong but could not say to him that such a thing could not be left for another day.
>
> The next morning testing showed the bilirubin level even higher. The physician on call reprimanded the nurse instead of the other physician.

A nurse too intimidated to speak up for a helpless newborn deserves a reprimand. She also deserves a desensitization program to help her overcome her pathological fear of doctors before it becomes fatal . . . for one of her patients.

Then there are times when the nurse must act in the best interest of a patient because a doctor refuses to do so. Although we always hope for the best, it is wise to be prepared for the worst. Here is one of the worst situations I have ever encountered:

> An ambulatory middle-aged man in respiratory distress came into the ER of our private local hospital with his wife. He did not have a local MD, and after the initial history, I placed a call to our front floor to see if any of the attending doctors were in the hospital.
>
> I was told that Dr. *K* was in the house, and they would tell him of the problem, and he would come back and see the patient. I made the patient comfortable and began talking with the family.
>
> Dr. *K* arrived, and his first question to the patient as he stood in the waiting room of the ER was "Do you have insurance?" The patient replied he did. He said he was employed by a local gas station that carried _____ insurance for their employees.
>
> Dr. *K* replied that that insurance wouldn't cover hospitalization and the medical "won't even begin to pay my bill!" With that he turned and left the ER.
>
> The patient and his wife looked at me. Then they left also.

The doctor's behavior is abominable. The nurse's behavior is inexcusable. More accurately, it is her lack of behavior that is inexcusable.

Caught up in this situation, most of us would be left standing with our mouths open. The doctor would be out of sight before we could gather our wits about us. The doctor got away, but the patient shouldn't have.

This dramatic example is excellent for role play. It helps nurses think on their feet and prepares them for some bad situations in advance. In workshops wonderful responses have emerged ranging from one earth-shattering bellow, "Freeze, Buster!" to an "Oh, boy, I've been waiting for something like this ever since I entered law school. Now let me see if I am quoting you correctly, doctor. . . ."

One acting nurse turned to the acting patient and said, "Thank goodness that quack didn't lay a hand on you. Now I'll get you a *real* doctor."

Another pantomimed picking up the telephone saying, "Hello, Security Department? There's a mad man impersonating Dr. *K*. Yes, he was just here in the emergency room. I think you will be able to catch him. He's wearing. . . ."

All kidding aside, if you were the responsible person, how would you get proper medical attention for this patient?

You Have the Right to be Human

I was faced with a situation a few months ago where I thought I was being assertive, but evidently did not come across that way. I had identified a key employee (male) as being alcoholic, after he was referred to me for evaluation by one of our executive vice presidents.

I reported back to the VP that he was alcoholic. The VP in turn spoke to another officer of the company, and then called me for a meeting to make a decision as to any action to be taken.

As we have a loose "Employee Assistance Program" and I am the resource person to contact, I was under the impression I would be handling this case. Instead, I was told they would counsel this man as I was a female (he would have trouble relating) and "just the nurse."

I maintained that I was qualified through many alcoholism courses and counseling courses and Rutgers Summer School. This meeting lasted 2 hours, and as I was confident in my abilities to handle the matter, I attempted to maintain an assertive manner, without being intimidated by the presence of the vice presidents.

It was concluded that they would counsel this man. They at-

121

tempted to do this for a few months without success and finally sent him to me. This man is now one of our key employees again. But if I perhaps had been more assertive, he would have received the proper treatment much sooner.

Here is a nurse who did everything right. She was professional, persistent, and prepared. It's not her fault that she is "female" and "just a nurse." That's part of her humanness.

Because of her success with this employee, I don't think those VP's will ever dismiss her so lightly again. She has earned the respect she needs to get future jobs done. This example is a triumph.

Isn't it sad she is still haunted by thoughts that she should have done more? She shouldn't have to apologize for being human. None of us should.

CHAPTER 11

Problem Solving

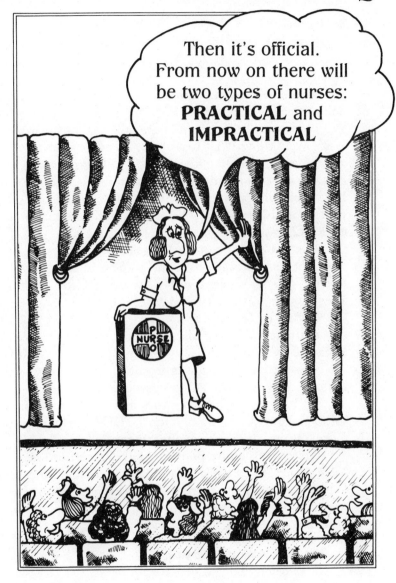

$\mathbf{T}$his is a dickens of a time to be in nursing. It is the best of times and the worst of times. On one hand, we seem to be making great strides toward autonomy. On the other hand, we are so confused we don't even know what to call ourselves.

Even if we could gather all 1.7 million nurses together and vote on the issues confronting us, we would never get a unanimous vote. If we wait for that impossibility to occur, problems will overrun our profession. It's not bad decisions that will undo nursing, it's the lack of decisions.

When I look back at my 20-year stint in nursing, I am dismayed to see the same problems cropping up again and again. I find consolation in Edna St. Vincent Millay's words, "Life is not one damn thing after another, it's the same damn thing over and over."

Writing in *The Courage to Create,*★ Rollo May discusses the painful contradiction of having to be fully committed yet all the while aware that we might possibly be wrong. He goes on to say that "the need for creative courage is in direct proportion to the degree of change the profession is undergoing."

Much of problem solving lies in having the courage to choose a solution from dissenting opinions. The heights we reach will depend more on our courage than anything else.

In effect this entire book is an exercise in problem solving. *Pro-Nurse Handbook* touches on problems ranging from procrastination to productivity, from recruitment to burnout, from exercising rights to facing responsibilities. This chapter is designed to help you solve problems not covered in the book. Here are:

Ten problem-solving tips
Think before taking action.

Be selective. Don't try to solve every problem that comes your
    way.

★May, Rollo: The courage to create, New York, 1976, W.W. Norton, Inc., p. 13.

Keep goal oriented.
Activate the 80/20 rule.
Make the best use of the world "as is."
Look for the opportunity hiding behind every problem.
Take the offense.
Learn to negotiate.
Make sure the solution matches the problem.
Expect success.

Think Before Taking Action

There are a half-dozen steps to most problem-solving attempts:

1. Define the problem (preferably in terms of need).
2. Generate a list of possible solutions.
3. Choose one.
4. Implement it.
5. Evaluate the outcome.
6. If the outcome is unsatisfactory, choose another solution or redefine the problem.

Here is a colorful example of the problem-solving process in action. A few years ago a dead whale washed up on the beach. The townspeople walked around the huge carcass trying to figure out how to dispose of it.

First, they tried to drag it back into the sea, but it was so heavy they couldn't budge it. Then someone suggested they cut the carcass into more manageable pieces. That sounded reasonable so they all rushed home to get their chain saws. Unfortunately, the saws just bounced off the whale's tough skin leaving barely a scratch.

By this time the carcass was beginning to decay. The people were becoming more desperate. Someone suggested they stuff the whale with dynamite and blow it apart. (*Moral: Desperate people are not responsible people.*)

Well, they dynamited the critter. It rained whale for miles. Do you have any idea how much damage a flying 20-pound chunk of decaying whale flesh can do?

When the air cleared, the townspeople really had something to blubber about. The bulk of the carcass remained intact on the beach, but now the landscape was splattered with putrifying fragments. (*Moral: Some solutions are worse than the problems.*)

Finally, they decided to send for some sort of derrick to hoist the whale up and drop it out over the ocean. While waiting for the big equipment to arrive, the tide came in and carried the carcass away. (*Moral: Time and tide wait for no derrick.*)

Be Selective—Don't Try to Solve Every Problem That Comes Your Way

Don't be overzealous when it comes to tackling problems. Pause. Make sure the problem is yours or that you are the optimal person to solve it.

Keep a close reign on your good intentions. If the problem actually belongs to someone else, you won't have the authority to enact a lasting solution, and if the problem's owner does not fully endorse your solution, failure is inevitable.

Providing solutions to someone else's problems is often a thankless task. The world is full of ungrateful little twits who will criticize rather than commend your efforts.

If at first glance it appears you are the *only* person willing or able to deal with a problem, look again. Something is amiss.

Practice conservation. Concentrate your efforts on the very few problems that really deserve or require attention. Many nurses find their own problems raging out of control because they diverted all their resources into solving other people's problems.

Keep Goal Oriented

Many nurses find themselves plunging headlong through one helter-skelter day after another. They find other people's schedules and priorities constantly override their own. They work hard but accomplish little. Their efforts consistently exceed their results.

These nurses are suffering from *goal deficiency,* an acute or chronic disease that has reached epidemic proportions. Symptoms include:

1. Indecision
2. Confusion
3. Frenzied activity
4. Lack of accomplishment

5. Desire to be told what to do and where to go
6. Growing resentment

At the onset of such symptoms, nurses have a tendency to step up their activity. Much like the oft-quoted observer of a bungled military operation said, "Having lost sight of our objective, we redoubled our efforts."

It's not the lack of effort but the lack of goals that keeps successes few and far between.

Basically you need two sets of goals: long haul and short run. Your long-haul goals reflect your life's grand plan. What grand plan? If you don't have one, grab pencil and paper and head for a quiet spot where you can do some uninterrupted thinking.

Write answers to the following questions:

1. What do I want to accomplish in my lifetime?

2. What do I want to be doing 2 years from now?

   Five years from now?

3. If these were my last 6 months on earth, how would I live them?

"What do I want to accomplish in my lifetime?"

Stumped? You may find it helpful to write your own fictitious obituary. Sometimes condensing your life's accomplishments and pleasures into a few paragraphs can help you decide whether to enroll in college or buy steamship tickets, volunteer to help the Red Cross or learn to tap dance, have a baby or run for political office.

Implicit in this issue is determining what you want to accomplish in your *professional* lifetime. You may need to change jobs or careers if your real obituary is to read properly.

"What do I want to be doing 2 years from now? Five years from now?"

A man wrote to an advice columnist saying he wanted to go to medical school but lamented the fact that he was already 35 years old. He worried that when he began his practice, a full 7 years from now, he would be 42 years old.

The columnist wrote back asking, "And how old will you be in 7 years if you don't go to medical school?"

All of us are getting older. Some of us are getting better. What about you? Are you spending time or investing it?

"If these were my last 6 months on earth, how would I live them?"

If you're leading a cluttered, crowded life and find it difficult to set priorities, try asking yourself the question posed by British critic F.L. Lucas, "Is it worth the amount of life it will cost?"

If you knew you had only 6 months left, I'll wager you would make a lot of changes. You would simply refuse to waste time and energy on people, places, or things that were unimportant.

The connection between daily activities and the sum total of life's accomplishments is easily lost. That's why it is so important to ask yourself these questions at regular intervals. Remember, what you do in the short run determines what you accomplish in the long haul.

In workshops I often ask nurses to write down one of their personal or professional goals. Most stare at their scratch paper, pens immobilized. "Come on," I coax, "just write down one thing that would make your personal or professional life more satisfying." When they still hesitate I ask them to write down something they *wish* were different in their personal or professional lives. That opens the flood gates. Wishes are so much easier to articulate than goals.

"I wish I were thinner!"
"I wish I had my degree."
"I wish I had more weekends off."
"I wish administration would listen to the nurses."
"I wish I were rich."
"I wish I could speak French."
"I wish I could be promoted."
"I wish I could find a husband."

"I wish I could take a trip around the world."

"I wish. . . ."

Because it's easier to be a dreamer than a doer, lots of nurses have dreams, but few have goals. What's the difference between a dream and a goal? A *workable* plan.

Many of us are reluctant to admit that making dreams come true has little to do with luck and lots to do with hard work: our own hard work and no one else's. "But let us learn if nothing else that hard work in the absence of goals and workable plans to achieve them remains just that—hard work."*

If you're tired of hard work that doesn't seem to be getting you anywhere, try this next exercise. Take a moment to compile your own wish list. Then select one of your fondest wishes and complete the following:

One thing I want that would make my *personal* or *professional* life

more satisfying is ————————————————— .

1. What do I need to do to get what I want?

2. What am I *willing* to do to get what I want?

3. How will getting what I want affect my life?

4. Who can I count on to help me get what I want?

5. What might I do to sabotage myself so I don't get what I want?

The key to achievement is developing a workable plan specific to each of your goals. For example, say I would like to lose 10 pounds.

---

*Hennig, Margaret, and Jardim, Anne: The managerial woman, New York, 1981, Doubleday & Co., Inc., p. 213.

What do I need to do? Cut calories and start exercising. What am I willing to do? Neither! Therefore, being thinner is a dream, not a goal. I am unwilling to do what is necessary.

It's that second question of what I am *willing* to do that separates dreams from goals, fantasies from realities. Nurses wish they were everything from medical missionaries to ballet dancers, but once they ask themselves the questions in this exercise, they quickly see how rare workable plans are. Most are unwilling or unable to do what it takes to make their dreams come true.

For years I've dreamed of owning a house on the Oregon coast. I grew up in Iowa, and when I saw the ocean, I thought I had died and gone to heaven.

Using this exercise I converted that dream into a goal. Today I have a workable plan that includes a special savings account and a subscription to the coastal newspaper. I have a realtor and am learning about the pros and cons of owning vacation property.

The third question is pivotal. "How will getting what I want affect my life?" If you appear to reach a dead end because you are unwilling to do what is necessary, this question may breathe new life into your dream or goal.

For instance, before abandoning my goal of losing 10 pounds, I asked myself how being thinner would affect my life. The benefits held great promise, so I pledged to undertake both diet and exercise.

(In the case of owning ocean property, this question may have the opposite effect. The responsibilities, risks, and realities of long-distance ownership may make a negative impact on my life. Turning my dream into a plan may help me to avoid turning my dream into a nightmare.)

"Who can I count on to help me get what I want?" After years of sedentary snacking, I didn't think I could count on myself to lose weight. That's why I enrolled in Weight Watchers and an aerobic exercise class. My husband rallied and joined me in both dieting and exercise.

Surrounding yourself with people who have similar goals increases your chance of success. Avoiding people who don't share your goals will also increase your chance of success. Look at the people who surround you at home and at work. Who can you count on? Who can you convert?

"What might I do to sabotage myself?" I may postpone getting started succumbing to the "someday syndrome." I may convince myself I am not really fat, I am just short for my weight. I may tell myself I am too busy to exercise. I may neglect my diet because the holidays are approaching or company is coming or any of a hundred other excuses.

This five-question exercise can be used for any of those wish list items nurses named: getting a college degree, speaking French, improving communications, getting a promotion, finding a husband, becoming rich, or taking a trip around the world.

Occasionally it's possible to achieve two goals with one plan. For nurses who want to be married and rich, Joanna Steichen, a psychotherapist in New York, teaches a course titled, "How to Marry Money." Her qualifications? She is the widow of a wealthy photographer who was 50 years her senior.

Workable plans—what do you need to do? What are you willing to do? How will your life be affected? Who can help you? How might you sabotage yourself?

This simple exercise can also help our profession delineate dreams from goals. For example, nursing wants to be accepted as a "profession." What does nursing need to do? It needs to develop an organized body of specialized knowledge, a code of ethics, standards of practice, consistent educational guidelines, a commitment to research, and peer review.

What is nursing *willing* to do? Therein lies the rub. To date nursing has been either unwilling or unable to meet society's minimal criteria for professions. A blatant shortcoming is in nursing's educational preparation. Professions require professional education that is normally above and beyond the baccalaureate level. So far nursing hasn't even risen to that lowest baseline: the baccalaureate degree.

Nursing educational problems have plagued us long enough. It's time to decide whether acceptance as a profession is worth the effort or not. Either way, making a decision will break us free to pursue goals instead of dreams.

Activate the 80/20 Rule

Long ago and far away, an Italian economist named Pareto spoke of an 80/20 rule. Loosely translated, his rule says that if all items or tasks are listed, 80 percent of the value, satisfaction, or results will come from 20 percent of the list.

For example, 80 percent of the sales come from 20 percent of the customers, 80 percent of the sick leave is used by 20 percent of the employees, 80 percent of the prescriptions repeat 20 percent of the drugs, and my own personal favorite, 80 percent of the dirt is on 20 percent of the floor.

It's true. Look at your kitchen floor. There is usually a distinct path of dirt. If you grab your mop and take a swipe down that path, in a couple of minutes your kitchen floor will be 80 percent cleaner. If you drop to your knees and wipe every inch of the floor, you will invest 80 percent more time but only increase the cleanliness 20 percent.

By learning 20 percent of the drugs, procedures, laboratory tests, diets, diseases, and interventions, students can acquire 80 percent of what they need to know. Of course, if you want to pass, you have to study the *right* 20 percent.

Generalists master the 20 percent that is applicable 80 percent of the time. Specialists master the additional 80 percent knowing full well they will only be using it 20 percent of the time.

If you have ten tasks to do for a patient, two of them will make 80 percent of the difference. When schedules are tight or tempers short, it is important to know which two those are.

Admitting we can't meet everyone's every need encourages us to concentrate on high-priority needs. Who determines which needs have highest priority? Each individual. That's why accurate, open communication is imperative.

If the doctor's highest priority is to get the patient's signature on the surgical consent form and he finds it undone, he will be irritated. The fact that all sorts of other good things were done for his patient will not appease him. If the patient desperately wants a shampoo but doesn't get it, he will complain about the lousy care at this hospital in spite of everything else done for him. If the nurse sees predischarge teaching as the most important thing for a particular patient but is unable to get around to it, she will leave work feeling frustrated. Her lack of accomplishment in that one area will obscure her many accomplishments in other areas.

The easiest way to determine priority is to *ask* those involved. One postpartum nurse gives her new parents a dozen index cards each with a different heading like feeding, bathing, immunizations, and the like. Couples then select topics they wish to have the nurse discuss with them. They leave the hospital raving about the personalized attention they received because *their* needs were met.

Imagine you find yourself working on a hospital unit that is fraught with problems. Morale is low and turnover high. Sometimes the sheer number of problems immobilizes people. Knowing you can't solve all the problems may keep you from solving any.

If you have ten outstanding problems, which one should you tackle first? *Ask!* Ask your co-workers, "If you could change just one thing on this unit, what would it be?" Listen closely and you'll find one or two problems consistently emerging as high priority. Solving the top two problems may improve morale so much that everyone is able to live with the other eight.

All too often management misreads employees' needs and priorities. They may spend lots of time and money correcting eight problems and only improve the situation 20 percent. They made a great effort. They just don't understand why they didn't get great results.

Efficiency experts help clients identify and concentrate on that 20 percent that yields an 80 percent return. Therefore, their clients can make wise investments whether in terms of time, money, personnel, or effort. Now you know their secret too.

Make the Best Use of the World "As Is"

If only taxes weren't so high . . .
If only the paint weren't peeling . . .
If only it didn't rain so much . . .
If only I had a child . . .
If only everyone would stop smoking . . .
If only doctors would respect nurses . . .
If only there were a college in town . . .

We've all played the if-only game. Some of us play it to excess. We spend all our time wishing things were different instead of working with things as they are.

Nurses who base their expectations and actions on a world as it *should be* or *ought to be* rather than on the world as it *is* are destined for frustration and failure.

Learn the system. Use it. It might not seem like much, but it's all we've got.

Look for the Opportunity Hiding Behind Every Problem

Listening to the president of one state's nursing association present their new nurse practice act, I was struck by her constant referral to the nurse as "he." For me, that's like listening to fingernails grating on a blackboard.

Nursing is a woman's profession—*97 percent female*. To deny that fact not only causes problems, it prevents us from seeing the opportunities.

Instead of cursing the difficulties presented by a predominantly female work force, think of the advantages. Women work harder, longer, and cheaper than men. They are more interested in relationships than reward or recognition. After the age of 45, a Metropolitan Life Insurance Company study showed that *male* employees registered more disability days than female employees. Many corporate studies have demonstrated that older female workers are more dependable, have low turnover rates, better attendance records, stay on the job longer, and do as much work as their younger counterparts. To top it all off, few women ever collect any pension benefits.

Of course, there are some problems associated with a predominantly female staff. One is that women still carry 90 percent or more of the responsibility for child care in our culture. Attitudes on this subject are changing, but behavior isn't.

When Child Care Systems of Cambridge, Massachusetts, surveyed employees at a large health care facility, they found up to 45 percent of the workers missed work, arrived late, or left early because of inadequate child care arrangements. An even more important finding was that *75 percent* were worried about the reliability of their present child care arrangements.★

That's a problem! The solution? Many corporations are sponsoring on-site child care. The benefits have far exceeded their expectations.

When the University of Wisconsin surveyed 58 organizations sponsoring child care, the employers reported a 57 percent reduction in turnover and a 72 percent decrease in absenteeism. Employee attitudes toward their employer improved dramatically along with their attitudes toward work. The companies sponsoring child care

---

★Casselberry Manuel, Diane: The tycoon and the toddler, Grad. Woman **76:**17, 1982.

also said it had improved community relations and stimulated positive publicity, and 88 percent reported the program had attracted new employees.

Over half the mothers of preschoolers are gainfully employed and their number grows daily. Two-income families are becoming the rule instead of the exception. When both mother and father are working, a sick child is more than an inconvenience, it can be a crisis.

Seeing both the problem and a profitable solution, Children's Hospital in St. Paul, Minnesota, developed a special child care service department. They dispatch licensed practical nurses and specially trained nursing assistants to care for sick children in their own homes. The charge is $4.00 an hour and available to anyone who needs it. Business is booming.

Take the Offense

Be a TOAD. That's an acronym for take offensive action, dummy!

Nice nurses reading this book will need reassurance that there is quite a difference between being offensive and taking the offense. Think about offense as it's used in sports. Teams alternate playing defense and offense.

In the game of life nurses have spent almost all their time on defense. We have struggled to keep other professionals from gaining ground on us. All the while the opposing players have been chanting, "Push 'em back, Push 'em back, *WAY* back!"

No wonder nurses haven't made many points. To score, we have to grab the ball and run. We have to play offensively.

There are some "offensive" nurses in Oregon—nurse practitioners who acquired prescriptive privileges and went into private practice. At first the physicians weren't very concerned. They expected the nurses to disperse among the rural poor. But some of those nurses had the nerve to open up offices right next door to the doctors in downtown Portland!

Most doctors would be surprised because that's not the sort of future they envision for nurses. A national cross section of physicians polled in a 1982 Harris survey said that by 1990 nurse practitioners and physician's assistants will have more responsibility for initial diagnosis and treatment of the rural and urban poor, children and pregnant women, the elderly, and the chronically ill.

135

Reading between the lines, physicians evidently see themselves caring for the rural and urban *rich,* adult men, nonpregnant women, the nonelderly, and the acutely ill. No offense, docs, but I'm getting tired of being expected to take care of your nonprofitable patients. If that sounds crass and flagrantly mercenary, it probably is.

Honestly, I am not advocating abandoning the young, old, poor, or chronically ill. I just want to emphasize that nurses need a financially healthy mix of patients every bit as much as those other health professionals do if we are to stay in business.

A nurse who is well compensated by eight of her patients can afford to donate her services to two who cannot pay for care. Unfortunately, nurses expect to eke out a living on two paying clients while donating their services to eight who cannot pay.

Nurses are always moaning, "But who is going to take care of the poor?" Why don't we ever moan, "But who is going to take care of the rich?"

Recently I met a man who asked himself just that. He opened a home health agency that caters to the well insured and well endowed. One client demands 'round-the-clock registered nurses for which she pays him $100,000 a year. The client doesn't *need* professional nursing care, but when you have $20 million in the bank, you can have whatever you want.

Currently this entrepreneur has four offices in a large city. In the next 5 years he plans to open 50 to 100 more around the country. He is a wheeler-dealer whose gutsy and unorthodox methods will either make him a millionaire or land him in jail.

The do-gooder in me just had to ask him about the poor people who couldn't afford such a service. He assured me he was sympathetic, but first and foremost he was a businessman. If he couldn't turn a profit, he couldn't stay in business long enough to take care of anyone.

A newspaper article titled, "Hospitals Can Make Money," quoted John Bedrosian, executive vice president of the eminently profitable National Medical Enterprises, Inc., a company that owns or operates over 200 hospitals and long-term care facilities.

Bedrosian says hospitals that fail to make a profit are mismanaged. They usually lack adequate inventory control, are not properly reimbursed by Medicare and Medicaid, and have poor controls on staffing. "You cannot have the luxury of too much nursing," he says.

". . . The luxury of too much nursing"—that phrase nearly leaped off the paper at me. Nursing as a luxury. I had thought of nursing as a need, a necessity, a right, a responsibility but never a *luxury*.

Could it be that we have missed our best bet: marketing professional nursing care as a luxury. Picture a commercial with a satisfied patient saying, "Sure, professional nursing care costs a little more, but *I'm* worth it."

Let's mount an offensive. Let's not wait for clients to come to us. Let's go for it! After all, "We're the most expensive nurses in America . . . and darn well worth it!"

Learn to Negotiate

The mark of a successful negotiation is that everyone leaves with some, if not all, of their needs satisfied. Nurses are just beginning to learn that almost everything in life is negotiable.

Here is a nurse who had a perfect opportunity to negotiate but muffed it:

> I was in the nursing office last week when our staffing coordinator was discussing a staffing dilemma with another nurse. I volunteered to work an extra night to help her out.
>
> Where I should have negotiated was the fact that I really wanted Saturday night off. I should have said, "I will work the extra night *if* I can have Saturday night off." Needless to say, I worked Saturday and Sunday and have the extra night to "look forward to."

In this situation both the coordinator and the staff nurse have needs. The staff nurse volunteers to meet the coordinator's need without even expressing her own need. Now she is kicking herself. She had everything to gain and nothing to lose by negotiating.

If she had made the offer and the coordinator saw it as a satisfactory solution, both would have been happy. If the proposed solution solved one problem but created another, namely a Saturday shortage, it may not have worked. Since the proposal was contingent on a mutual satisfaction of needs, the staff nurse can gracefully withdraw saying, "It was just a suggestion. I'm sorry we couldn't work something out."

Nurses are so used to meeting others' needs while ignoring their own that they lack experience in negotiating. Supervisors, used to having nurses volunteer with no strings attached, may be surprised as nurses gain some sophistication in negotiating skills.

Negotiations can range from getting one night off to collective bargaining for the whole institution. When negotiations break down, the ultimate solution is a strike. Many think a strike would be more correctly called the ultimate problem.

Strike! Few nurses are comfortable with that solution . . . or problem.

For years we have labored under the delusion that a nurses' strike would leave patients dying in the streets. But do you know what happens when doctors go on strike? The mortality *drops!* The most plausible explanation is that elective surgery is postponed and patients are sent home. (We all know a hospital is the worst place to be if you're sick.)

In actuality, a nationwide nurses' strike might save thousands of lives. Patients are in more jeopardy when nurses passively continue to work in spite of broken equipment, inadequate supplies, inept doctors, and a staff that is tired, ill-prepared, or inexperienced.

Make Sure the Solution Matches the Problem

Remember, implementing a solution is not the last step in the problem-solving process. Before you can lay the problem to rest, you have to evaluate the outcome. That evaluation determines whether a problem is truly solved or whether it needs to be reworked.

Nursing has an abundance of problems: unwieldly work loads, compressed salaries, inconsistent educational policies, subordinate status, subservient mentality, little respect, lack of autonomy, responsibility without authority, and relatively few opportunities for advancement—real or otherwise.

Perfectly good solutions for one problem are totally worthless when applied to other problems. Take advanced education. Although it may be a solution for some of the above problems, it is not a solution for all of those problems.

At a national meeting one irate nurse demanded to know just when her education was going to pay off. She had felt pressured to acquire her bachelor's and master's and was now working on her doctorate. Along the way she felt she had been promised the solution to nursing's economic problems could be found in education. That promise was proving false, and she was mad as a hornet.

If you think education will improve your financial status, think again. At every point in the life cycle a male high school graduate will make more than a college-educated female. For 20 years the difference in average educational attainment between men and women has only been one tenth of a year. Men earn twice as much as women because they invest in a different type of educational capital. Women still invest in fine arts, teaching, nursing, and other social and service-oriented fields.

Another nurse who had recently completed her PhD found herself more than $10,000 in debt. For her sacrifice and accomplishment, she received a $500 a year raise. With luck she will recoup her investment before she retires.

If she had counted on advanced education to solve her financial problems, she would be as angry as the other nurse. Although the piddling monetary gain disappointed her, she found her education would "pay off" in other ways. She was enjoying her new status, increased autonomy, unsolicited job offers, and opportunities for recognition in her specialty area. Education solved some of her problems, and happily, they were the problems she found most pressing.

Expect Success

Our actions and our beliefs are inextricably intertwined. It's not the truth per se but what we *believe* to be true that guides our behavior. If we expect success, we will move steadily toward it. If we expect failure, we will move steadily toward that.

What you believe to be true about yourself is vitally important because every moment you move toward making your self-image a reality. Do you see yourself as marginal or magnificent? Intelligent? Decisive? Energetic? Creative? Successful? Respected? Professional?

Whether the adjectives you use to describe yourself are positive or negative, your actions will be directed toward making them accurate. That makes it wise to accentuate the positive and eliminate the negative.

The same holds true for the nursing profession. Our profession is also moving steadily toward making its collective self-image a reality. Is the image of nursing marginal or magnificent?

If you alter your beliefs about yourself or nursing, a change in behavior will occur. You can actually trick yourself into changing for better, for worse, for richer, for poorer, toward sickness, or toward health.

Behaviorists, of course, contend it is much easier to alter behavior than beliefs. They contend acting differently will bring about a compatible change in beliefs.

For example, if you want to appear confident, walk 25 percent faster. People will think that you are a person who really knows where she is going. As you walk along at a faster clip, you will actually begin to feel more confident. Soon you are a person who really knows where she is going.

To *survive,* you have to call a halt to self-defeating beliefs and behaviors. To *thrive,* you have to replace them with positive thoughts and actions.

STOP	START
Putting yourself in jeopardy— physically, mentally, emotionally, financially	Taking care of yourself— physically, mentally, emotionally, financially
Trying to rescue *everyone* (especially those who do not wish to be rescued)	Helping others accept responsibility for their own actions and problems
Dreaming	Planning
Wishing for good things	Working toward goals
Apologizing for what you are not	Rejoicing in everything you are
Conforming	Creating
Wishing others were more thoughtful or helpful	Asking for what you want and need
Trying to be *Supernurse*	Delegating
Fretting	Enjoying
Being defensive	Taking the offensive
Wasting your time, talent, and energy	Investing your time, talent, and energy
Taking orders	Taking command
Agonizing over how things *should* be	Making the best use of the world "as is"
Believing in magic	Believing in yourself

More than leaders, nursing needs cheerleaders. Nursing needs positively-focused professionals who dare to raise their sights far beyond the survival threshold. Nursing needs professionals who want to thrive.

Pro-Nurse
"Do-It-Yourself" Epilogue

Where will you wind up?

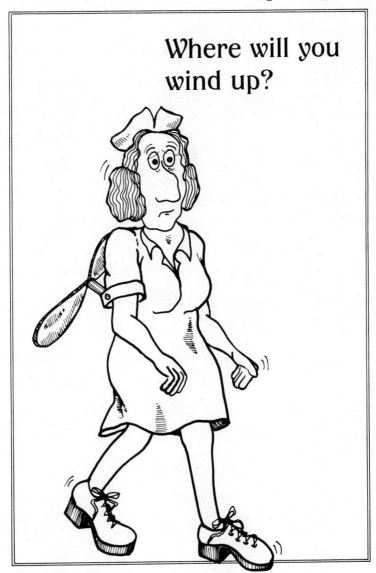

All wound up and no place to go? Wishing that someone would point you in the right direction so you'd be all set?

Well, I can wind you up, but no one can point you in *the* right direction. There are all sorts of right directions. You have all the pain and pleasure of choosing your own.

Picking the right direction is only possible when you know where you want to go. It might help to think of your life as a short story and take Edgar Allan Poe's approach. He wrote the endings first. Then he worked backward so they came out as he desired.

Write your ending first. Make it grand. If you keep the end in sight, making decisions along the way is much less complicated. Remember, the heights you reach will depend more on your courage than your ability.

Where will you wind up?

It's your choice. Dare to make it.

Index